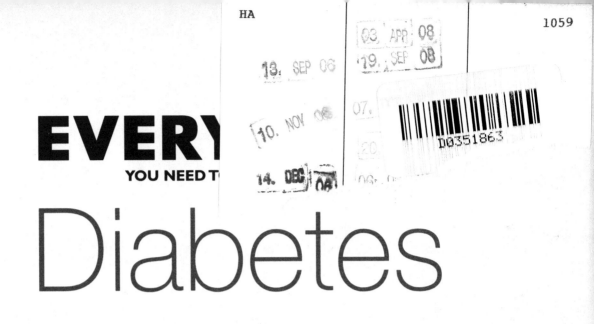

EVERY
YOU NEED T

Diabetes

EVERYTHING

YOU NEED TO KNOW ABOUT...

Diabetes

PAULA FORD-MARTIN

WITH IAN BLUMER, M.D.

David & Charles

A DAVID & CHARLES BOOK

David & Charles is a subsidiary of F+W (UK) Ltd.,
an F+W Publications Inc. company

First published in the UK in 2004

n the USA as The Everything® Diabetes Book,
dams Media Corporation in 2004

endments copyright © 2004 David & Charles
ht © 2002 Adams Media Corporation

No part of this publication may be reproduced,
al system, or transmitted, in any form or by any
or mechanical, by photocopying, recording or
e, without prior permission in writing
from the publisher.

Project Manager Ian Kearey
Cover Design Ali Myer

A catalogue record for this book is available from the British Library.

ISBN 0 7153 2057 2

Printed in Great Britain by CPI Bath
for David & Charles
Brunel House   Newton Abbot   Devon

Visit our website at www.davidandcharles.co.uk

David & Charles books are available from all good bookshops;
alternatively you can contact our Orderline on (0)1626 334555 or
write to us at FREEPOST EX2110, David & Charles Direct,
Newton Abbot, TQ12 4ZZ (no stamp required UK mainland).

Contents

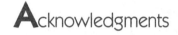Acknowledgments

My heartfelt thanks to Ian Blumer, MD, whose knowledge, experience and terrific sense of humour made writing this book a pleasure. And to those who made writing it a privilege – thanks to Marcie, Andrea, Harvie, Sandi, Char, Bev and all the other 'regulars' at the About Diabetes forum. Your courage, compassion and insight have helped so many – including me. Finally, thanks to Barb Doyen and Eric Hall, encouragement and patience personified.

Top Ten Things You Should Know
About Diabetes

1. Eating sugar does not cause diabetes. And contrary to popular belief, people with diabetes can eat sugar in moderation, as long as it's considered in their overall meal plans.

2. The terms 'insulin-dependent' (Type 1) and 'non-insulin-dependent' (Type 2) diabetes are inappropriate. People with Type 2 diabetes do require insulin sometimes.

3. Adults can develop 'juvenile' (Type 1) diabetes, and children can develop 'adult-onset' (Type 2) diabetes.

4. Having 'a touch' of diabetes is like being 'a touch' pregnant. There is no such thing as borderline diabetes.

5. There is no 'diabetic diet', only a new, healthier way of eating.

6. Learning as much as you can about diabetes and consulting a registered dietician are two of the most important ways you can start controlling your diabetes.

7. People with diabetes can work out and play sports. Exercise lowers blood glucose levels and is an important component of good diabetes management.

8. Diabetes is not a death sentence, but it can lead to serious, life-altering and life-threatening complications if ignored.

9. Checking yourself frequently with a home blood glucose monitor can help prevent blood glucose emergencies, and the monitor is an invaluable tool for learning how food and medication affect your disease.

10. People with diabetes – both adults and children – are protected against discrimination in the workplace and at school by a number of laws introduced in the Disability Discrimination Act (1995).

Introduction

▶ IF YOU'VE PICKED UP THIS BOOK, the chances are that diabetes has touched your life or the life of someone close to you. Whatever the manifestation – Type 1, Type 2 or gestational – diabetes can be a frightening and personally devastating diagnosis. Fortunately, patient knowledge and action are probably the two most important components in staying on top of this disease.

A key phrase in the lexicon of diabetes care is *good control*. For those new to the topic, good control means keeping your blood glucose in a range at or close to normal through diet, exercise and/or medication. Control is the key to managing diabetes mentally as well as physically. The power is in your hands to make a difference in how diabetes affects your life.

Many people feel out of control of their diabetes. Some ignore it completely in a fog of denial. Others follow medical instructions to the letter, yet never ask questions of their doctor or provide any feedback. The latter may get a handle on their blood glucose levels, but they are so miserable it hardly matters.

Managing diabetes requires education, dedication and a certain doggedness of character. Most important, it requires a commitment to being a leader, not a follower, in your own health care. Surrounding yourself with good people – diabetes specialists, diabetes specialist nurses, registered dieticians, podiatrists and more – is an excellent start. But it takes more than a top medical team to control diabetes. Even the best team will falter without a leader, and that leader is you. Playing an active role in your own health care is essential to staying both healthy and happy.

Uncontrolled blood glucose levels wreck havoc on the body, damaging just about every system over time if not managed properly. Heart disease, stroke, high blood pressure, eye disease, kidney disease and nerve damage are just a few of the complications that diabetes leaves in its wake. This is why educating yourself about the intricacies of glucose control – through diet, exercise, medication, lifestyle and more – is essential.

Medical breakthroughs, such as islet cell transplantation, advances in glucose monitoring technologies and new oral medications and insulin formulations, have drastically improved the quality of life for all people with diabetes, but there is still no cure for the disease. Until there is, keeping up to date on developments in diabetes management, communicating with your health care team, and staying on top of self-care through positive lifestyle choices are absolutely essential to being well. This book is designed to be your reference partner in staying healthy with diabetes.

Chapter 1

What is Diabetes?

Diabetes mellitus comes in many forms – Type 1, Type 2, gestational and variations such as maturity-onset diabetes in the young (MODY) and latent autoimmune diabetes of adulthood (LADA). What all of these disorders have in common is an inability to self-regulate the levels of blood glucose – or cellular fuel – in the body.

A Growing Problem

More than 1.4 million people in the UK have been diagnosed as having diabetes – that's at least 3 per cent of the population. In addition, there are thought to be at least 1 million more people who have diabetes, although they don't know it yet since it hasn't been diagnosed. This figure is projected to rise to 3 million by 2010, as levels of obesity rise and the population ages. Worldwide, numbers are also escalating and diabetes is fast becoming a global health problem.

Type 2 diabetes accounts for around 90 per cent of the total diabetes population in the United Kingdom. However, moderate levels of regular physical activity and a healthy diet can reduce a person's chance of developing Type 2 by up to 60 per cent.

In addition to the personal physical and emotional problems caused by diabetes, it also comes with an enormous price tag, picked up by the NHS. The total cost of diabetes care in the UK is thought to exceed £2 billion, and this is set to double during the next decade. Diabetes accounts for about 9 per cent of hospital costs – and the hospital costs for a person with diabetes are thought to be six times higher than for a person without diabetes. It isn't just diabetes that is running up the bill; much of the economic burden is related to long-term complications of the disease.

The Endocrine System

Diabetes mellitus is classified as a disease of the endocrine system. The endocrine system is composed of glands that secrete the hormones that travel through the circulatory system to regulate metabolism, growth, sexual development and reproduction. When one of these pivotal glands – the adrenals, the thyroid and parathyroid, the thymus, the pituitary, testes, ovaries and the pancreas – secretes either too little or too much of a hormone, the entire body can be thrown off balance.

The Pancreas and Liver

One of the endocrine glands, the pancreas, also works as a digestive organ. Sitting behind the stomach, the spongy pancreas secretes both digestive enzymes and endocrine hormones. It is long and tapered with a thicker bottom end, which is cradled in the downward curve of the duodenum – a part of the small intestine or bowel. The long end of the pancreas extends up behind the stomach towards the spleen (see figure on page 5). A main duct, or channel, connects the pancreas to the duodenum.

While the term 'diabetic' is a useful adjective for describing things and conditions related to diabetes – diabetic supplies, diabetic kidney disease, etc. – many people with the disease bristle at being labelled 'a diabetic'. People with diabetes should not have to be defined by the disease, nor marginalized because of it.

Pancreatic Tissues

In the pancreas, specialized cells within the *exocrine* tissue secrete digestive enzymes into a network of ducts that join the main pancreatic duct and end up in the duodenum, where they are vital in processing carbohydrates, proteins and other nutrients.

The *endocrine* tissues of the pancreas secrete hormones from cell clusters known as *islets of Langerhans*, named after Dr Paul Langerhans, who first described them in medical literature. Islets (pronounced EYE-lets) are comprised of three cell types:

- **Alpha cells** manufacture and release glucagon, a hormone that raises blood glucose levels.
- **Beta cells** monitor blood glucose levels and produce glucose-lowering insulin in response.
- **Delta cells** produce the hormone somatostatin, which researchers believe is responsible for directing the action of both the beta and alpha cells.

Another Key Player: The Liver

Located towards the front of the abdomen and above the stomach, the liver is the centre of glucose storage. This important organ converts glucose – the fuel that the cells of the human body require for energy – into its principal storage form, *glycogen*. Glycogen is stored in muscle and in the liver itself, where it can later be converted back to glucose for energy with the help of the hormones adrenaline (secreted by the adrenal glands) and glucagon (from the pancreas).

Some people with Type 1 diabetes keep an emergency glucagon injection kit at hand. Glucagon is a hormone that prompts the liver to release glycogen and convert it into glucose. It is used to treat a severe hypoglycaemic episode (severe low blood sugar) in Type 1 or Type 2 diabetes.

Together, the liver and pancreas preserve a delicate balance of blood glucose and insulin, produced in sufficient amounts to both fuel cells and maintain glycogen storage.

Insulin and Blood Sugar

While the liver is one source of glucose, most glucose the body uses is derived from food, primarily carbohydrates. Cells then metabolize, or burn, blood glucose for energy. Insulin is the hormone that makes this all happen.

To visualize the role of insulin in the body, we can use a lock and key analogy. Imagine that for glucose to enter a cell, a door must first be unlocked. Insulin is the key that is needed to unlock the door and let the glucose in. In this analogy, the insulin receptor on a cell is the door, and the important part of this is that which binds the insulin; i.e., the lock that the key must fit.

There may be lots of glucose in the bloodstream, but without insulin to bind to the cell receptors (no keys that fit the locks on the doors), the glucose cannot enter cells to be processed. Instead, the glucose builds up to damaging and toxic levels in the bloodstream, while the body's cells are deprived of their energy source.

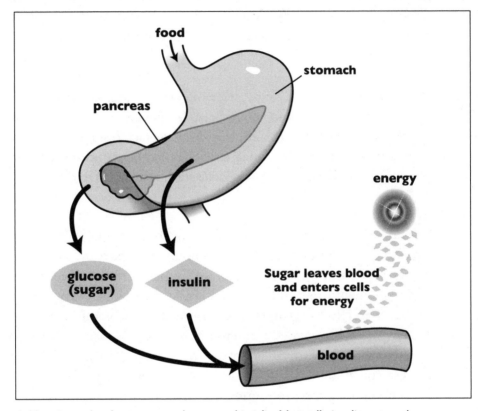

▲ How it works: the pancreas, glucose and insulin. Normally, insulin enters the bloodstream to regulate the levels of glucose.

What Goes Wrong in Diabetes

In people with Type 1 diabetes, the key is missing (no insulin production), or there are only one or two needles to fit an entire mansionful of locks (insufficient insulin production). This happens when the islets (specifically the insulin-producing beta cells) of the pancreas are destroyed. In people with Type 2 diabetes, the key is either not a good fit, or, sometimes, the lock itself is a faulty one. This latter phenomenon, where there's plenty of insulin but the body isn't using it properly, is known as *insulin resistance*. It also occurs in gestational diabetes mellitus (GDM), a type of diabetes that starts in pregnancy. Some people with Type 2 diabetes go on to develop a certain amount of beta cell death and insulin insufficiency as well (not enough keys made). Gestational diabetes usually resolves itself after childbirth, although women who develop GDM have a higher risk for developing the permanent insulin resistance of Type 2 diabetes later in life.

Although the name is almost the same, diabetes insipidus (also known as *water diabetes*) is a condition completely different in cause and treatment to diabetes mellitus. Diabetes insipidus is characterized by a problem with the kidneys that impedes their ability to concentrate urine adequately, usually due to a deficiency in antidiuretic hormone (ADH).

The human body needs glucose to function, but too much glucose circulating in the bloodstream has the potential to be toxic, a problem known as *glucotoxicity*. When insulin isn't available, blood glucose levels rise higher and higher in the bloodstream. Fatigue, excessive thirst, increased urination and flu-like symptoms such as nausea and vomiting may appear. A severe rise in blood glucose can result in diabetic ketoacidosis (DKA) or hyperglycaemic hyperosmolar nonketotic coma (HONK), sometimes called diabetic coma – both are life-threatening medical emergencies.

A timely diagnosis and immediate treatment are important in preventing DKA, HONK and other complications. In the long term, elevated blood glucose levels can damage virtually all the systems of the body. Blood vessel damage can result in cardiovascular disease, nerve damage, retinal eye disease, nephropathy and more. To learn more about preventing complications, see Chapter 15.

Managing Diabetes: a Balancing Act

While chronically high glucose levels are the hallmark of diabetes, blood glucose levels that dip too low are also a hazard of the disease. Hypoglycaemia, or a low blood glucose level, is dangerous because the central nervous system requires glucose to function properly. The most common triggers for a 'hypo' are:

- An imbalance of food and insulin, such as when too much insulin is administered for the amount of carbohydrates eaten.
- Exercise without sufficient carbohydrate intake.
- Excess alcohol intake.

Some people also experience night-time dips in blood glucose levels as their liver shuts down glucose production during sleep.

Controlling Blood Glucose

The ultimate goal of management of any type of diabetes is to keep the blood glucose level as close to normal as possible. The charity Diabetes UK suggests that people with diabetes aim for blood glucose levels of 4–7 mmol/l (millimoles of glucose per litre of blood) before meals and no higher than 10 mmol/l after meals.

It's important to remember that each patient has unique glucose goals. Those who are very susceptible to episodes of hypoglycaemia may have a slightly higher baseline goal than those who aren't, while women who are trying to bring their glucose levels down as part of a pre-conception plan for pregnancy may have a lower baseline for tighter control. Your doctor or diabetes specialist nurse will work to determine what goals are right for your particular medical history and lifestyle.

A normal non-fasting blood glucose reading in a person without diabetes would usually be between 3.5 and 8 mmol/l. A random plasma glucose reading of 11.1 mmol/l or higher, a fasting plasma glucose reading of 7.0 mmol/l or higher, or an oral glucose tolerance test with a two-hour postload reading of 11.1 mmol/l or higher are high readings that may indicate diabetes.

Treatment Tools

How do you bring blood glucose levels down to a controlled range? Each person will have his or her own unique treatment plan, but the main tools at your disposal are diet, exercise and medication. People with Type 1 diabetes require insulin therapy. Those with Type 2 diabetes can sometimes control their diabetes with a combination of dietary regulation and exercise, while others may require some oral medication and/or insulin. No matter what your type of diabetes, proper nutrition and exercise should be a cornerstone of both diabetes management and healthy living.

The Name Game

Diabetes is the Greek word for 'siphon' (since people with uncontrolled diabetes tend to urinate copiously). *Mellitus* is Latin for 'honey' or 'sweet'; this name was added when physicians discovered that the urine from people with diabetes is sweet with glucose.

Long before the advent of diagnostic urine testing in the 19th century, one of the earliest ways that physicians used to make a diagnosis of diabetes was to taste a patient's urine.

As researchers began to understand diabetes more, different subtypes of the disease were classified. Type 1 diabetes was once routinely called insulin-dependent diabetes mellitus (or IDDM), and Type 2 diabetes was called non-insulin-dependent diabetes mellitus (NIDDM). The problem with this classification scheme was that it defined diabetes not by the cause of the disease, but by its treatment – specifically, whether or not a patient required insulin injections. This was often confusing because so-called non-insulin-dependent (Type 2) patients do frequently require insulin therapy.

Types and Subtypes of Diabetes	
Classification	**Includes these clinical subtypes**
Type 1	Type 1A (LADA)
	Idiopathic Type 1B
Type 2	N/A
Gestational	N/A
Other types, caused by the following:	Genetic beta cell defects (like MODY)
	Genetic insulin action defects
	Other genetic syndromes
	Diseases of or injury to the pancreas
	Other endocrine disorders
	Drugs or toxins

For more information on particular types and subtypes of diabetes, read Chapters 2 and 3.

Also confusing was the system of calling Type 1 diabetes 'juvenile diabetes' and Type 2 diabetes 'adult-onset diabetes'. While most cases of Type 1 diabetes are diagnosed in childhood and adolescence, adults of any age, from 20-something to the elderly, can develop the disease. In recent years, Type 2 diabetes has begun to appear in younger adults and children as obesity rates soar. In short, there are no age limits to either type of diabetes.

In the late 1990s, the World Health Organization recommended using Type 1 diabetes and Type 2 diabetes as the clinical standard to explain these very complex, similar yet completely different diseases. However, you may come across a few medical people, and many laypeople, who still use the old names and terms.

Chapter 2

Type 1 Diabetes

Type 1 diabetes, also previously called juvenile diabetes, childhood diabetes or insulin-dependent diabetes mellitus (IDDM), occurs when 90 per cent or more of pancreatic beta cells have been destroyed, usually by an autoimmune process that impels the body to attack itself. Consequently, the body produces little to no insulin. Without insulin to assist in processing, glucose in the blood rises to damaging and potentially fatal levels.

Type 1A, or Autoimmune, Diabetes

Although there are several different subtypes of Type 1 diabetes, the most common form of Type 1 diabetes is an autoimmune disease, or an attack from within. For some reason, the body's immune cells don't recognize the beta cells of the pancreas as part of the body, and instead attack them as if they were foreign invaders. The trigger behind this autoimmune siege is not completely understood. Current research points to a combination of environmental and genetic factors.

Certain diseases that damage the pancreas (such as haemochromatosis, cystic fibrosis and pancreatitis) may cause beta cell destruction that can eventually lead to diabetes and insulin dependence. In addition, some endocrine disorders, including Cushing's syndrome and acromegaly, cause hormone imbalances that influence the way insulin is produced and processed by the body, subsequently leading to diabetes.

Signs of Self-Destruction

An antibody is a protein that works along with other immune system components to destroy a specific foreign presence in the body, such as bacteria or a virus. An autoantibody is an antibody gone haywire – it attacks cells in the body that it is supposed to protect.

Up to 90 per cent of individuals with Type 1 diabetes test positive for the presence of islet cell antibodies (ICA), insulin autoantibodies (IAA) and/or autoantibodies to glutamic acid decarboxylase (a beta cell protein known as GAD). These autoantibodies attack and destroy the insulin-producing beta cells. A positive islet cell antibody test can actually detect the autoimmune processes that attack the beta cells of the pancreas before clinical symptoms of hyperglycaemia (high blood glucose levels) actually occur. When Type 1 diabetes is known to be caused by an autoimmune process, it is referred to as *Type 1A* diabetes. Immune-mediated Type 1 diabetes also puts you at a higher risk for developing other autoimmune disorders, such as coeliac disease, thyroid disease, myasthenia gravis and others.

Latent Autoimmune Diabetes in Adults

A subcategory of Type 1A diabetes, latent autoimmune diabetes in adults (LADA), occurs in approximately 10 per cent of all cases of diabetes in adults over the age of 30. This immune-mediated form of diabetes is sometimes referred to as late-onset autoimmune diabetes in adults, slow-onset Type 1 or Type 1.5 diabetes. Basically, individuals with LADA experience a slower and longer process of beta cell destruction than those with classical Type 1A diabetes.

Type 1B, or Idiopathic, Diabetes

Type 1B diabetes is also referred to as *idiopathic diabetes*, or diabetes of unknown origin. This form of Type 1 diabetes is not autoimmune in nature, and tests for islet cell antibodies will come up negative.

Some people with Type 1B have an absolute insulin deficiency and are prone to ketoacidosis. This form is more common among people of African and Asian origin. In another form, found more commonly in Africans, the insulin requirement typically waxes and wanes, and these people may periodically experience ketoacidosis.

Genetics and Heredity

Exactly what sets off the complex mechanisms behind beta cell destruction and eventual insulin dependence is not completely understood, but researchers believe it is likely that a genetic predisposition to the disease activated by an environmental trigger.

Genetic Markers

Human leukocyte antigens (HLA) are a set of surface blood proteins that help to control immune function. Two specific HLA markers – HLA-DR and HLA-DQ – help the immune system to identify foreign invaders, and have been specifically linked with type 1A diabetes.

However, while everyone with Type 1 diabetes is thought to have an example of these genetic markers, not everyone with a marker goes on to develop diabetes. For this reason, genetic testing can be helpful in identifying the possibility of diabetes but not in determining with certainty that it will occur.

How do I know if I have Type 1A or Type 1B diabetes?
The issue is largely an academic one. The expense and scarcity of autoantibody tests at this point in time makes them impractical for routine use, and knowing your type probably won't have any real bearing on the course of treatment. The overall approach to disease management is the same, and even some Type 1B individuals may have some periods of insulin independence.

In addition to statistical uncertainty, it is also cost-prohibitive to use genetic testing to screen for Type 1 diabetes, and because there are no known methods of delaying or preventing the disease if a genetic tendency is revealed, the test serves no practical purpose. However, in circumstances where it is unclear if a patient is Type 1 or Type 2 and early diagnosis may provide a way to preserve some degree of islet cell function, testing may be appropriate.

Family History

Heredity is a relatively small piece of the puzzle in predicting Type 1 diabetes. Statistically, people with an immediate family member who has Type 1 diabetes are 15 times more likely than the general population to develop the disease. Yet only 10 per cent of people with Type 1 have a first-degree relative with the disease.

Having a parent with Type 1 places you at an approximate 5 per cent risk of developing the disease (2–3 per cent for the mother and about 6 per cent for the father). If you have a sibling with the disease, your risk is an estimated 6 per cent.

Looking at cases of Type 1 in identical twin studies puts the role of heredity in an even better perspective. In cases where one identical twin develops Type 1 diabetes, an estimated 30–70 per cent of their twin siblings will develop it. In other words, having a carbon copy gene set of someone with diabetes isn't a guarantee that the disease will occur. Something in the environment must flip the switch.

Ethnicity

In the UK, Type 1 diabetes tends to be more common in the Caucasian population. On a global scale, both geography and ethnicity play a part in the rates of diabetes among certain populations. For example, Finland and Sardinia (Italy) have the highest incidences of Type 1 diabetes worldwide, while Asian countries like Japan and China have extremely low rates of the disease.

A good way to remember the core difference between Type I and Type 2 diabetes is in terms of insulin processing. People with Type I diabetes are insulin-*deficient*, meaning their pancreas is producing little to no insulin. In contrast, most people with Type 2 diabetes initially generate enough insulin, but because they are insulin-*resistant*, their bodies can't use it to process blood glucose.

Environmental Triggers

What exactly triggers the autoimmune system to self-destruct beta cells is not clear, but studies have implicated several viable theories. Environmental toxins, a virus or a medication may be the final physiological straw for someone genetically predisposed to the disease.

By 2003, clinical studies had implicated 14 different viruses in beta cell damage and the development of Type 1 diabetes, including adenovirus, coxsackie B virus, mumps virus, enteroviruses, rubella virus, cytomegalovirus and Epstein-Barr virus.

It's important to remember, however, that developing one of these viruses does not necessarily mean that you will develop Type 1 diabetes; specific genetic programming for the disease must also be present.

Cow's Milk

Exposure to cow's milk and cow's milk-based formula before one year of age has been associated with the development of Type 1 diabetes in some studies, although other research has found no link. Study results are also mixed on the role of dietary proteins and their association with the development of autoimmunity and Type 1 diabetes in both animal and human trials. In 2002, the Juvenile Diabetes Research Foundation, the National Institutes of Health and several other governmental and advocacy organizations in the USA announced a large-scale, multinational study called TRIGR (Trial to Reduce Insulin-Dependent Diabetes in the Genetically at Risk). TRIGR was designed to be the first large-scale, long-term study to assess the relationship of infant formula consumption in relation to the likelihood of developing Type 1 diabetes in infants considered genetically at risk for developing the disease. The two-year study has involved 6,000 families in 14 countries, including the UK, and will hopefully determine with certainty the association, if any, between Type 1 diabetes and milk proteins.

Clinical research has found that babies who breastfeed for at least three months have a lower incidence of Type 1 diabetes, and may be less likely to become obese as adults.

Other Causes of Beta Cell Destruction

Certain toxins, drugs, genetic defects and diseases of the pancreas can also cause beta cell destruction, leading to diabetes mellitus. The occurrence of diabetes in this category is relatively rare – and as such, their causes and specific treatments are not covered in this book.

Signs and Symptoms

Physical signs of Type 1 diabetes usually appear rapidly as uncontrolled high blood glucose, or hyperglycaemia, reaches crisis levels. Symptoms include the following:

- Excessive thirst
- Frequent urination
- Extreme hunger
- Unexplained weight loss
- Fatigue, or a feeling of being 'run down' and tired
- Rapid breathing
- Blurred vision
- Dry, itching skin
- Headaches
- Tingling or burning pain in the feet, legs, hands or other parts of the body
- High blood pressure
- Mood swings, irritability and depression
- Frequent or recurring infections, such as urinary tract infections, yeast infections and skin infections
- Slow healing of cuts and bruises.

A blood plasma glucose test, either random (any time of day) or fasting (no food or drink eight hours prior), is usually used to diagnose Type I diabetes. If symptoms are present, and the blood test reading is high, then diabetes may be diagnosed immediately. Otherwise, a second test on a different day may be performed to confirm the diagnosis. Turn to Chapter 6 to read about these tests in detail.

Diabetic Ketoacidosis (DKA)

When blood glucose levels are extremely high (persisting in the teens), signs of DKA may also start to appear. Ketoacidosis is life-threatening and requires immediate medical attention. Symptoms of DKA include those listed overleaf.

- Lethargy
- Nausea and vomiting
- Abdominal pain

· Fruity breath smell
· Rapid breathing
· Dehydration
· Loss of consciousness.

DKA is also diagnosed by the presence of ketones in the urine. (For more on urine testing for ketones, see Chapter 6.)

Hyperosmolar Nonketotic Coma (HONK)

Individuals with Type 1 diabetes can also develop a condition known as hyperosmolar nonketotic coma (HONK), which is characterized by many of the same symptoms as DKA, and usually occurs when blood sugar levels are about 30 mmol/l, without ketoacidosis. However, HONK is rare in Type 1 diabetes, and occurs more frequently in people who have Type 2 diabetes.

Insulin is Not a Cure

Subcutaneous injections of insulin are the frontline treatment for Type 1 diabetes. However, it's important to realize that insulin is not a cure for diabetes, nor can insulin treatment erase the potential for complications and increased risk for other autoimmune disorders that accompany the disease. The only current 'cure' for the disease is the transplantation of a healthy, functioning pancreas or of insulin-producing beta cells, and even that procedure is not without its own set of risks and potential problems (see Chapter 22).

The finely tuned internal biological mechanisms that dispense just the right amount of insulin in response to blood glucose levels are absent in Type 1 diabetes patients. While injected exogenous insulin (insulin produced outside the body) can bring blood glucose levels down to a safe level, it is a far from perfect system. The type and amount of insulin and the timing and location of injections are just a few of the many factors that influence how well the treatment works. The dose of insulin must adequately cover the amount of carbohydrates that will be eaten and the corresponding rise in blood sugar levels. Too much insulin, and hypoglycaemia (or low blood glucose) results. Too little, and blood glucose levels rise too high. Precision is important, yet can be elusive.

Children and adults diagnosed with Type I diabetes sometimes experience a period of remission known as the 'honeymoon period', which usually occurs shortly after diagnosis as blood glucose levels are brought under control. During a 'honeymoon', the remaining islets are functioning sufficiently and the need for insulin injections is greatly reduced, or sometimes even eliminated completely.

Vigilant attention to diet, a good understanding of how changes in carbohydrate intake affect insulin dose, and basic maths skills are essential to proper treatment; yet, even with these, insulin can often be a game of chance. Circumstances such as emotional stress, use of other medications and even something as seemingly simple as the common cold can result in skyrocketing blood glucose levels and a potential diabetic emergency. For more on insulin treatment, see Chapter 8.

Chapter 3

Type 2 Diabetes

Type 2 diabetes, the most common type of diabetes, is also one of the most prevalent chronic diseases around. Worldwide, more than 150 million people suffer from it; the International Diabetes Federation projects that this population will double globally by 2025. While weight is a major risk factor for Type 2 diabetes, ethnic background, family history and certain other components of your health profile also play an important role.

Insulin Resistance and Type 2

As with Type 1 diabetes, Type 2 diabetes is a metabolic disorder in which blood glucose rises because it isn't being effectively balanced and metabolized into cell energy by insulin. The similarities in physiology between the two types end there, however.

Type 2 diabetes is not caused by the absence of the hormone insulin, as is the case with Type 1, but rather by the body's inability to use insulin properly. People with Type 2 have a condition called insulin resistance. They can produce insulin, usually in sufficient amounts at first, but it doesn't bind properly to the insulin receptor that is the gateway to cells in muscle, fat and liver tissue, and they are therefore resistant to its effects. In other words, it's like trying to fit a square peg (insulin) into a round hole (insulin receptor). As a result, glucose doesn't enter the cells and instead builds up in the bloodstream, resulting in high blood sugar levels.

The causes of Type 2 diabetes are complex and not completely understood, although research is uncovering new clues at a rapid pace. Animal studies have associated certain genetic markers with the development of the disease, and its relationship with obesity has become clearer in recent years.

The second condition that sets the stage for Type 2 diabetes is insulin deficiency – the pancreas also has difficulty producing sufficient amounts of insulin to process the rising blood glucose levels. Eventually, it does not have sufficient amounts to overcome the deficit. The toxic effects of long-term high glucose levels on the insulin-producing beta cells of the pancreas (glucotoxicity) can make insulin deficiency worse.

Some people with Type 2 are highly insulin-resistant with a small amount of related insulin deficiency. Others are primarily insulin-deficient and just slightly insulin-resistant.

'Prediabetes'

Sometimes a person's blood glucose level is a little higher than normal, but not high enough to be officially diagnosed with diabetes. 'Prediabetes' is a term that is increasingly being used to describe this scenario. In clinical terms, the condition may be impaired fasting glucose (IFG) or impaired glucose tolerance (IGT), depending on the type of blood glucose test performed. IFG is diagnosed if the result of a fasting blood glucose test is between 6.1 and 7.0 mmol/l. IGT is diagnosed if the result of a glucose tolerance test is between 7.8 and 11.1 mmol/l.

Not all people with IFG or IGT go on to develop Type 2 diabetes; however, these people are at risk of developing Type 2 diabetes and related complications, especially heart disease.

One of the reasons for the boom in Type 2 diabetes is the widening of waistbands and the trend towards a more sedentary lifestyle. People with 'prediabetes' may be able to delay, or perhaps prevent, the onset of Type 2 diabetes by making lifestyle changes such as losing weight and becoming more active.

Progression to Type 2 Diabetes

The pancreas of a person with Type 2 diabetes generates insulin, but the body is unable to process it in sufficient amounts to control blood glucose levels. In some cases, this is due to the chemical make-up of the insulin itself, but most of the time it is connected to how the body's cells – specifically the insulin receptors that attract and process the hormone – recognize and use insulin. As blood glucose levels rise, the pancreas pumps out more and more insulin to try to compensate. This may bring down blood sugar levels to a degree, but also results in high levels of circulating insulin, a condition known as hyperinsulinaemia. At a certain threshold, the weakened pancreas cannot produce enough insulin; in some cases, insulin secretion is actually reduced by the toxicity of high glucose levels to pancreatic beta cells. At this point, Type 2 diabetes results.

While most people with Type 2 diabetes have some degree of insulin resistance, not everyone with insulin resistance has Type 2 diabetes. Metabolic syndrome X is a constellation of symptoms – insulin resistance, low HDL and high LDL and triglycerides, excess abdominal fat and high blood pressure – that puts you at risk for heart disease.

Risk Factors

The biggest indicator for your risk of Type 2 diabetes is the diagnosed presence of IFG or IGT. But since the vast majority of people with 'prediabetes' remain undiagnosed, assessing the presence of the other common risk factors for Type 2 diabetes is important.

Age

Type 2 diabetes tends to occur in adults over the age of 40, and the risk increases with age, so that the older you are, the greater your risk is.

Obesity

Being overweight is probably the most important risk factor for developing Type 2 diabetes; over 80 per cent of people with Type 2 diabetes are overweight. The more overweight you are, the greater your risk of diabetes. There is more detailed information on obesity and related factors in the next section of this chapter.

Reduced Physical Activity

A sedentary lifestyle can contribute to diabetes in its own right, as well as by increasing the tendency towards being overweight. Building up the level of physical activity can decrease the risk of developing Type 2, independently of age or weight.

Ethnicity

Certain ethnic groups in the UK have a greater risk of developing Type 2 diabetes. Afro-Caribbean and Asian people are four to five times more likely to have diabetes than Caucasians.

Family History

Heredity plays a significant part in the development of Type 2 diabetes. As a general rule, it seems that the closer the family relative, the greater the risk is. If you have a first-degree relative who is affected, then your chances of developing Type 2 are doubled. There is a concordance rate of up to 90 per cent among identical twins with Type 2, meaning that where one twin has the disease, the other twin has a 90 per cent chance of developing it as well.

Hypertension

Having high blood pressure (greater than 140/90 mmHg – millimetres of mercury pressure) is a risk factor for the development of Type 2 diabetes, as well as being a possible complication of the disease.

Blood lipid profile and cholesterol levels

Low levels of HDL cholesterol and high levels of triglycerides in the blood increase the risk of developing Type 2 diabetes, in addition to a predisposition towards heart disease.

Gestational Diabetes

Women who have had gestational diabetes (GDM) during pregnancy are at an increased risk of developing Type 2 diabetes; statistically, between 20 and 50 per cent of women with a history of gestational diabetes go on to develop Type 2 within five to ten years of giving birth.

Birth Weight

Giving birth to a baby weighing over 4kg (9lb) is considered a risk factor for later development of Type 2 diabetes in the mother.

Women who have a history of gestational diabetes should be mindful that they may develop Type 2 diabetes at some stage in later life and be on the lookout for signs and symptoms. Regular blood glucose checks by the GP are important so that diabetes is caught early on, before serious complications develop.

Risk Associated With Weight and BMI

According to a report published by the UK National Audit Office, the prevalence of obesity in England has almost trebled over the past two decades. Currently, over half of women and about two-thirds of men are either overweight or obese (see opposite for definitions of these terms). In total, one in five adults is obese.

Being overweight or obese is a primary risk factor for developing Type 2 diabetes and associated complications.

Why is Weight a Risk Factor?

Too much fat makes it difficult for the body to use its own insulin to process blood glucose and bring it down to normal circulating levels. Why? There are three reasons:

- **Overweight people have fewer available insulin receptors.** When compared to muscle cells, fat cells have fewer insulin receptors, the place where the insulin binds with the cell and 'unlocks' it to process glucose into energy.
- **More fat requires more insulin.** The pancreas starts producing larger and larger quantities of insulin in order to 'feed' body mass, and consequently insulin resistance turns into a catch-22 situation. Excess

blood sugar must be stored as fat, and excess fat promotes further insulin resistance.

· **Fat cells release free fatty acids (FFAs).** Fat cells and tissue, particularly abdominal fat, release free fatty acids, which interfere with glucose metabolism.

Leptin, a hormone in fat cells that helps to metabolize fatty acids, has provided an important clue to the relationship between obesity and Type 2 diabetes. Discovered by researchers at Rockefeller University, USA, in 1995, leptin (named after the Greek *leptos*, meaning 'thin') also plays a part in sending a satiety – or 'all full' – signal to the brain to stop eating when body fat increases, and an 'empty' signal when body fat is insufficient. It appears that a type of leptin resistance may lead to a situation where fatty acids are deposited instead of metabolized, leading to eventual insulin resistance.

Your BMI

Obesity and body fat are measured by body mass index (BMI) – a number that expresses weight in relationship to height and is a reliable indicator of overall body fat. You can calculate your BMI as follows:

$$BMI = (Weight\ measured\ in\ kilograms)/(Height\ measured\ in\ metres)^2$$

The World Health Organization (WHO) defines as 'overweight' people with a BMI of 25–30 and as 'obese' those with a BMI of more than 30. People with a BMI of more than 40 are described as being severely or morbidly obese. At least 80 per cent of people with Type 2 diabetes are overweight or obese at diagnosis.

Defining obesity in children and young adults is more complicated, as BMI changes substantially with age. A charting system called BMI-for-age compares each child's weight in relation to other children of the same age and gender on a growth chart in terms of percentiles. However, there is as yet no international consensus on the appropriate cut-off points, although a standard definition has been proposed based on international data.

You know smoking is bad for your health, but did you also know that it can increase your diabetes risk? Smoking constricts blood vessels, raising blood pressure and increasing the risk of coronary artery disease. It also stimulates the release of catecholamines, which have been shown to promote insulin resistance.

Body Shape

Although BMI is a useful index, it doesn't take the distribution of body fat into account, and this is an important factor when it comes to insulin resistance. Having an apple-shaped body, with excess pounds packed around the waist (as opposed to a pear-shaped body, with large hips) is an independent risk factor for insulin resistance and Type 2 diabetes. According to the World Health Organization, a waist circumference exceeding 94cm (37in) for men, or 80cm (31½in) for women, confers an increased risk for health problems.

Signs and Symptoms

Both Type 1 and Type 2 diabetes exhibit the same basic symptoms of hyperglycaemia. Some symptoms, such as tingling or burning in the hands and feet (neuropathy), are the result of long-term uncontrolled blood glucose, and are more common in Type 2 patients. It's important to note that not all people with Type 2 diabetes will have symptoms, particularly in the early stages of the disease. In fact, up to a third of all people with type 2 diabetes are unaware that they have it.

Symptoms of Type 2 diabetes may include one or more of the following:

· Thirst and frequent urination
· Dry, itching skin
· Headaches
· Tingling or burning pain in the feet, legs, hands or other parts of the body
· High blood pressure

· Mood swings (such as irritability or depression)
· Fatigue, or a feeling of being 'run down' and tired
· Blurred vision
· Extreme hunger
· Unexplained weight loss
· Frequent or recurring infections (e.g. urinary tract infections, yeast infections)
· Slow healing of cuts and bruises.

 Women of reproductive age who have developed polycystic ovarian syndrome (PCOS) are at an increased risk for Type 2 diabetes. PCOS is a hormonal disorder characterized by enlarged ovaries containing fluid-filled cysts. Women with PCOS have irregular menstrual cycles and high circulating levels of male hormones (like testosterone). Insulin resistance and impaired glucose tolerance are manifestations of PCOS.

Hyperosmolar Nonketotic Coma

When blood glucose levels exceed about 30 mmol/l, a condition known as hyperosmolar nonketotic coma (HONK) may occur. In HONK, the body becomes severely dehydrated and fluids are depleted from the bloodstream. Older adults tend to develop HONK more readily, although the condition can occur at any age.

HONK is life-threatening and requires immediate medical attention. Symptoms of the syndrome include:

· Dehydration
· Excessive thirst
· Nausea and vomiting
· Fever
· Hypotension (low blood pressure that may be signalled by dizziness or faintness)

- Disorientation
- Sudden excessive sleepiness
- Seizures
- Visual disturbances and/or hallucinations
- In extreme cases, coma or hemiplegia (paralysis or weakness on one side of the body).

Hyperinsulinaemia

Hyperglycaemia is not the only abnormality to be found in Type 2 diabetes. As glucose levels build up in the bloodstream, the pancreas puts out more and more insulin in an effort to bring them back down. Consistently high levels of circulating insulin result in a condition known as *hyperinsulinaemia*.

People with Type 2 can also develop diabetic ketoacidosis (DKA), but it is not as common as it is in Type 1 diabetes, and generally occurs only as a result of a major physical stressor, such as a heart attack.

Diagnosing Type 2 Diabetes

A blood plasma glucose test, either random (at any time of day) or fasting (no food or drink for eight hours beforehand), is usually used to diagnose Type 2 diabetes. A normal, non-fasting blood glucose reading is about 3.3–7.8 mmol/l. A random plasma glucose reading of 11.1 mmol/l or higher, a fasting plasma glucose reading of 7.0 mmol/l or higher, or an oral glucose tolerance test with a two-hour postload value of 11.1 mmol/l or higher are high readings that may indicate diabetes. For more on diagnosing diabetes, see Chapter 5.

Long-term uncontrolled blood glucose levels can cause major damage to virtually every system in the body, from head to toes. If you experience any of the symptoms of diabetes, it's crucial to visit a doctor as soon as possible for evaluation. If a diagnosis is made, maintaining tight control of your blood glucose levels is the best way to avoid serious complications.

Maturity-onset diabetes in the young (MODY) is a group of rare forms of diabetes caused by specific genetic defects. Although MODY is treated like Type 2 diabetes, with diet, exercise and occasionally oral medications, it is a distinctly different class of diabetes.

Not Just for Adults Anymore

Type 2 diabetes, which was once considered an 'adults-only' disease, is now appearing in children and teenagers. A recently published study estimated the prevalence of Type 2 diabetes in children as 0.21/100,000. That figure equates to about one in every 500,000 children. 92 per cent of the children with Type 2 diabetes were obese. The same study reported that South Asian children in the UK have a relative risk of Type 2 diabetes of 13.7 compared to white children in the UK.

The incidence of Type 2 diabetes in children in the UK is still relatively low; however, it is set to become more prevalent with increasing rates of childhood obesity being reported. Today's children tend to live a far more sedentary lifestyle, centred around passive entertainment mediums like television and video games. In addition, the growth of the fast-food industry has integrated high-calorie foods into our children's society. In the UK, estimates of obesity in children range from 6 per cent in preschoolers to 17 per cent at 15 years of age.

Children at Risk

The self-same factors that place adults at great risk for Type 2 diabetes apply to children as well, and obesity is far and away the primary threat in this age group.

Acanthosis nigricans (darkening of the skin) is present in up to 90 per cent of children and adolescents who develop Type 2 diabetes. This condition is a clinical sign of insulin resistance and is more common in people with darker skin pigmentation. The dark, velvety patches typically appear in areas where skin folds gather – usually on the neck, armpits and groin – and are associated with high levels of circulating insulin (hyperinsulinaemia).

Having a family history of Type 2 diabetes among first- and second-degree relatives, and being of ethnic minority origin also increase the likelihood that overweight children will develop the disease.

The majority of childhood Type 2 cases are diagnosed at puberty or beyond. Puberty itself is the cause of a certain degree of insulin resistance in adolescents, which is thought to be triggered by a natural rise in growth hormone during this time. In children who are already disposed towards the disease, insulin resistance remains even after growth hormone returns to normal levels.

Treating Children for an Adult Disease

Diagnoses of Type 2 diabetes in children are sometimes difficult to make, especially in children who are not greatly obese. Many doctors still consider Type 2 diabetes an adults-only disease. It can present the same way as Type 1, with DKA or, in extreme cases, HONK. Often because of the age of the patient, Type 1 is initially suspected and the child begins insulin treatment. However, long-term use of insulin after blood glucose levels have stabilized can contribute to further weight gain, which can worsen the problem.

Children diagnosed with Type 2 diabetes can usually be treated through a combination of diet and exercise. Oral medications may be helpful, but clinical data is limited on their long-term effects in children.

My daughter is overweight, but we have no history of diabetes in our family. Should I really be concerned about her weight?

Yes. Weight problems in childhood can lead to the development of a host of medical problems, like atherosclerosis, hypertension, respiratory infections, sleep apnea and Type 2 diabetes. Talk to your doctor about a weight-loss strategy. And remember, diet and exercise should become a family affair to ensure the greatest chance of success for your daughter.

Chapter 4

Gestational Diabetes

Gestational diabetes, also known as gestational diabetes mellitus or GDM, is diabetes that is developed by women during pregnancy. It occurs in 2 to 4 per cent of pregnancies in the UK. Some women with GDM will go on to develop Type 2 diabetes later in life; it's been estimated that having GDM in pregnancy increases your Type 2 risk by up to 50 per cent.

Diabetes, Your Baby and You

Gestational diabetes is similar to Type 2 diabetes in that both are caused by a phenomenon known as *insulin resistance*. People who are insulin-resistant can produce insulin, but either their insulin receptors prevent it from binding correctly and allowing glucose to enter the cell, or, less commonly, there is something wrong with the insulin itself that makes it unable to work.

The placenta that is feeding your baby produces hormones, including oestrogen, cortisol and human placental lactogen, which work to counteract insulin. The result is a rise in blood glucose levels. In most pregnant women this rise is inconsequential, but in those who have developed significant insulin resistance, it grows to unmanageable levels and GDM results.

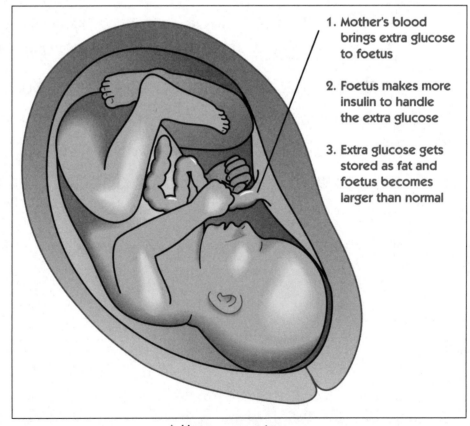

1. Mother's blood brings extra glucose to foetus

2. Foetus makes more insulin to handle the extra glucose

3. Extra glucose gets stored as fat and foetus becomes larger than normal

▲ How macrosomia occurs.

A Danger to You and Your Baby

Uncontrolled high blood glucose is damaging to both you and your baby. Over time, it can damage your nervous system, contribute to cardiovascular problems, impair your kidney function and make you more vulnerable to infection. It can also increase your risk of developing high blood pressure, and possible pre-eclampsia, in pregnancy.

High fasting blood glucose levels have been associated with an increased risk of foetal death in the final eight weeks of pregnancy. GDM also increases the risk of developing macrosomia, which can complicate delivery and has the potential to result in a birth injury.

Because your diabetes can cause your child's lungs to develop at a slower rate, she is at risk for respiratory distress syndrome, a condition in which inadequate production of surfactant (the substance that enables the alveoli, or air sacs, of the lungs to expand) makes breathing difficult for your baby after she is born.

Who is at Risk?

Your age, ethnicity, weight and medical history are all factors in your risk for developing gestational diabetes. You are considered at an increased risk for gestational diabetes if any one or more of the following risk factors apply:

- You are from a high-risk ethnic background – particularly Asian or Afro-Caribbean.
- You're overweight (as defined by a body mass index, or BMI, of 25 or higher).
- You have a first-degree relative with diabetes.
- You're over 25 years old.
- You have a history of GDM.
- You have a history of impaired glucose tolerance.
- You have had a baby weighing 4kg (9lb) or more in a past pregnancy.

At present there is no universal consensus on the screening for gestational diabetes. However, all pregnant women have their urine tested for glucose, usually at each antenatal visit, and random or fasting blood glucose levels are also checked periodically. Women with a high risk of gestational diabetes are likely to be screened more frequently.

Gestational Diabetes Diagnosis

The first sign that you've developed gestational diabetes may be glycosuria, or the sudden appearance of glucose in your urine. Virtually every pregnant woman spills a small amount of glucose into her urine, but if your doctor detects significant glycosuria during a routine urine test, she may order a plasma glucose test to measure the level of glucose in your blood. A level of 7.0 mmol/l or higher if you had been fasting at the time of the blood test, or 11.1 mmol/l or higher if you were not, points to hyperglycaemia (high blood sugar) and gestational diabetes.

An oral glucose tolerance test (OGTT) is frequently performed when screening for diabetes in pregnancy, and may be performed even if a fasting blood glucose result is less than 7.0 mmol/l. Gestational diabetes is diagnosed if blood glucose levels read 7.8 mmol/l or above, 2 hours after a 75g glucose load (you will probably be given Lucozade to drink). The OGTT is described in full in Chapter 5.

What to do First

If you are diagnosed with gestational diabetes, one of your first tasks will be to meet up with a diabetes specialist nurse (DSN) and a state registered dietician in order to develop a treatment plan and diet regime (you may be referred to a specialist antenatal-diabetic clinic at your local hospital). In addition to teaching you about blood glucose testing and other basics of managing your gestational diabetes, they can help you with strategies for dealing with morning sickness and other unique challenges of pregnancy. You will probably also have a consultation with a doctor who has special expertise in diabetes.

Treating Gestational Diabetes

To lower your blood glucose levels and minimize chances of complications for both you and your baby, you may need to make some lifestyle changes, including carefully watching what you eat and staying active.

Learning dietary control of gestational diabetes is a challenge because you have a short amount of time to learn what you need to know, and you need results fast. But pregnant women are what doctors like to call 'highly motivated patients'. That means that, like most mothers, you'll do just about anything to ensure your baby has the best possible start in life. So you start blood testing in earnest, learn the lingo of carbohydrate counting and read volumes on diabetes care.

A good diabetes specialist nurse and dietician are worth their weight in gold when it comes to learning about food and gestational diabetes. They will explain the basics of carbohydrate counting and coach you on the intricacies of portion estimates, good restaurant choices, your specific caloric and nutrient needs as a pregnant woman, and more. It also helps to have a good reference book or two around to consult. Chapters 10 and 11 explain these issues and healthy eating for diabetes in detail.

It's reassuring to know that many women with gestational diabetes are able to control their glucose levels through diet and exercise alone, but it's often that second word – exercise – that throws women into a panic. You should know that anything that gets your heart pumping and your body moving is good, and can lower blood glucose levels. That could be as simple as working in your garden or playing with your daughter at the park. If you need motivation, many health clubs, community centres and hospitals offer prenatal exercise classes.

For those who like a more solitary form of fitness, walking is a good way to ease yourself into a workout routine. It's cheap, easy and always accessible. Even if you live in an inhospitable climate for outdoor walking, you can find a local shopping centre or an indoor track to lap. If you've always been active, then you may be given the green light to do something a little more challenging. Always talk to your doctor first before starting any new fitness activity during pregnancy.

Monitoring Your Blood Glucose

Checking your blood glucose levels frequently with a portable home blood glucose meter is also an important part of your treatment programme. This quick and simple test involves pricking your finger with a fine needle, called a lancet, and placing a small blood drop on a test strip that is inserted into the meter. The meter analyzes the amount of glucose in the blood sample and displays the reading. (Chapter 7 has more information on how and when to test your blood glucose levels.)

Although the thought of 'pricking yourself' repeatedly is a deterrent to many when they first start checking glucose levels, keep in mind that with today's ultrafine lancets, the procedure is relatively painless. If you're experiencing a lot of pain or are having trouble getting a blood sample, take your meter and your technique to your diabetes specialist nurse (DSN), who can offer you pointers on less painful testing. You may be interested in trying a new meter or lancing technique – ask your DSN what's available.

When you first get started, you may be testing yourself more frequently as you try to get a handle on how different foods and activities affect your glucose levels. Testing is usually recommended early in the morning before breakfast (fasting test) and after meals (postprandial test). Postprandial tests are taken one hour after the start of your meal, and can be taken again at the two-hour mark. You should keep a written log of all your results (see Chapter 7 for a sample log page). If you exercise regularly, test your glucose levels before and after your workout.

Blood Glucose Target Levels in Women With Gestational Diabetes as Recommended by Diabetes UK	
Test	**Range**
Before meals	
Capillary whole blood glucose	≤5.6 mmol/l
Before meals	
Capillary plasma glucose	4.4–6.1 mmol/l
2 hours after meals	
Capillary whole blood glucose	≤7.8 mmol/l
2 hours after meals	
Capillary plasma glucose	≤18.6 mmol/l

Ketone Testing

In addition to blood glucose monitoring, your doctor may ask you to perform ketone testing at home. This is done by dipping a ketone test strip in a urine sample. Home blood glucose meters that also check for blood ketones are available. Ketones can be a sign that your blood glucose is too high and your body is breaking down fat stores for energy instead of glucose. They can also occur in cases of severe morning sickness if you aren't keeping adequate food down. If you test positive for ketones, call your doctor or DSN straight away for further directions.

When You Need Insulin

If you're unable to keep your blood glucose levels down to a safe level with dietary and activity changes only, your doctor may suggest insulin therapy. Oral medications aren't recommended because of the possible risks to the foetus, but insulin does not cross the placenta and is therefore safe for you and your developing baby.

Diabetes UK care recommendations for gestational diabetes advocate regular intake of low glycaemic index carbohydrates (see chapter 10), restricted intake of saturated fat and sugar, and a cautious reduction of calories if overweight. They suggest that insulin may be needed if pre-meal blood glucose readings exceed 6.0 mmol/l. Insulin may also be needed if the growth of the foetus (measured by ultrasound) is abnormal.

Another trip back to the DSN may be in order to teach you how to take insulin and to learn the signs and symptoms of hypoglycaemia (low blood sugar). He or she can also work with you to help you understand how to interpret your blood glucose readings and manage your insulin accordingly. Always bring your blood glucose log with you on both your antenatal and diabetes clinic appointments so you don't have to rely on your memory and so your health care team have a more accurate clinical picture on which to base treatment decisions.

Needing to take insulin does not mean you've 'failed' at managing your diabetes. Consider it another method of ensuring your baby the best possible birth outcome.

How Gestational Diabetes Affects the Baby

Just like babies born to mothers with Type 1 or Type 2 diabetes, newborns from mothers with gestational diabetes can experience hypoglycaemia at birth. Low levels of calcium and magnesium in your baby's blood may also be a problem. Jaundice, a yellowing of the skin that happens when your baby has excess bilirubin in his system, may also occur in babies born to mothers with gestational diabetes.

Fortunately, all of these conditions are usually easily correctable. And the fact that your diabetes has been diagnosed means that your health care team can anticipate these possible problems and diagnose and treat them quickly. You may also have a specialist paediatric doctor, or neonatologist, who treats high-risk infants, in the delivery room, or on stand-by, to care for your baby.

We had our 'birth plan' all worked out and ready to take to the midwife, but now that I've got gestational diabetes I'm wondering if there's any point?

Having gestational diabetes doesn't mean that all your wishes are automatically thrown out of the window. A written agenda of what you want during your labour and delivery may be even more important when you know interventions may be required. Your doctor and midwife can work with you to adjust your plan to reflect appropriate expectations. To learn more about birth plans, check *Everything You Need to Know About Pregnancy*, also in this series.

Foetal Macrosomia

Foetal macrosomia, or a baby who is too big for its term, can occur in women with gestational diabetes if their blood glucose levels aren't well controlled. Since your blood glucose crosses the placenta and passes into the foetal circulation, your baby will start to produce more and more insulin to counteract its effects. Even the most active baby can't burn off all that glucose (there's only so much room to move around in there). As a result, the extra glucose is stored as fat.

If an ultrasound reveals that your foetus is substantially big for the date, macrosomia may be suspected. If your child develops macrosomia, she may become too large to fit through the birth canal, and a caesarian section may be required. This is another reason why good control of your gestational diabetes is so important during pregnancy.

There are also risks to the health of both mother and child if the pregnancy continues right up to or over the full 40 weeks of gestation. For this reason, some obstetric teams like to induce labour at or around the 39th week. Talk to your doctor early about her thoughts on these interventions to work towards a birth experience that's acceptable for both of you and promotes the best possible outcome for your baby.

Beyond Pregnancy

After you've delivered, you'll have to remain vigilant about your and your child's health. When you visit your doctor for your postpartum evaluation, your glucose levels will once again be tested. If the results indicate impaired glucose tolerance (IGT or prediabetes), you will need to be tested in the future for diabetes.

Long-Term Risks to Mum

Having gestational diabetes increases the risk in subsequent pregnancies, and also increases your long-term risk of developing Type 2 diabetes. The good news is that the nutritional skills and exercise habits you pick up are your best defence against Type 2 diabetes, and your doctor will encourage you to continue to use them after delivery. Studies have shown that minor lifestyle changes and weight loss can make a big difference in lowering your insulin resistance.

Another thing you learned in pregnancy – awareness of highs and lows – should not be forgotten after the baby's birth. Remember what high blood glucose levels felt like, and if you ever develop the symptoms, see your doctor immediately.

If and when you decide to become pregnant again, schedule a preconception consultation with your doctor to assess your health status, have yourself screened for diabetes, and ensure that you get your next pregnancy off to a good start.

Is it OK to breastfeed after gestational diabetes?
Yes! In addition to all the known benefits that breastmilk and nursing offer your baby, breastfeeding may actually kickstart your pancreas, improving beta cell function and lowering your risk of developing Type 2 diabetes. Breastfeeding also burns extra calories (about 800 daily) and can help you lose excess pregnancy weight.

Long-Term Risks to Baby

Your new healthy lifestyle should also be something that carries over to your family life. Your child will be at an increased risk for obesity and diabetes as she grows into adolescence and adulthood. The best way to help her counteract this is to encourage and model good habits now that will last a lifetime.

Chapter 5

Diagnosis and Beyond

A diagnosis of diabetes is a scary thing, but having a health care team that is knowledgeable and communicative can make the ride a little less bumpy. Your doctor is only one part of the equation in diabetes – because diabetes is a systemic disease, you'll also be seeing a team of specialists to help prevent and treat complications. Play an active and educated role in your care, and you'll be in charge of your diabetes, rather than the other way around.

Making the Diagnosis

Diabetes is diagnosed through a lab test that measures the level of glucose in your blood. Because a rise in blood sugar levels might be attributable to some other factor, such as illness or stress, a second blood test may be performed the following day to establish the diagnosis.

There are actually three different types of diagnostic blood tests in use: the fasting plasma glucose test; the random plasma glucose test; and the oral glucose tolerance test. In the absence of overt symptoms or a hyperglycaemic crisis, two tests taken on different days are recommended to confirm the diagnosis.

Fasting Plasma Glucose Test (FPG)

The FPG is a test that measures plasma (blood) glucose levels after a fast of at least eight hours. Fasting stimulates the release of the hormone glucagon, which in turn raises plasma glucose levels by triggering the breakdown of glycogen (stored glucose) in the liver. In people without diabetes, the body will produce and process insulin to counteract this rise in glucose levels. With diabetes, this does not happen, and the tested glucose levels will be high.

The fasting plasma glucose test should be performed early in the morning. Blood glucose tests given in the afternoon tend to provide lower readings and could miss some cases of IGT and diabetes.

Diabetes UK recommend that the World Health Organization (WHO) criteria are adopted in the diagnosis of diabetes. According to WHO, a fasting reading of 7.0 mmol/l or higher indicates diabetes. In the absence of symptoms, a second test on a different day should be performed to confirm the diagnosis.

The normal range for the FPG is considered under 6.1 mmol/l. Individuals with FPG results between 6.1 and 7.0 mmol/l, or a two-hour glucose level rising to 7.8–11.0 mmol/l, are said to have impaired glucose tolerance (IGT) or impaired fasting glucose (IFG),which is sometimes referred to as prediabetes.

Random Plasma Glucose Test (RPGT)

The RPGT can be performed at any time of the day, regardless of whether the patient has eaten or not. Random plasma glucose levels of 11.1 mmol/l or higher, along with symptoms of diabetes, is considered diagnostic of diabetes. In the absence of symptoms, a second test on a different day should be performed to confirm the diagnosis.

Guidelines for Diagnosing Diabetes in the UK, based on World Health Organization (WHO) criteria			
Test	Normal Levels	'Prediabetes'*	Diabetes**
Fasting Plasma Glucose	<6.1 mmol/l	≥Impaired Fasting <Glucose 6.1–7.0 mmol/l	≥7.0 mmol/l
Random Plasma Glucose	<		≥11.1 mmol/l
Oral Glucose Tolerance Test	<7.8. mmol/l	Impaired Glucose Tolerance 7.8–11.1 mmol/l	≥11.1 mmol/l (2h postload)

*This term is currently not officially recognized by Diabetes UK
** In the absence of symptoms, a second test on a different day should be performed to confirm the diagnosis.

After a diagnosis is made, further lab tests may be ordered to determine the progression of your disease and the possibility of coexisting conditions that are common in diabetes.

Oral Glucose Tolerance Test (OGTT)

The OGTT is a test that measures blood glucose at hourly intervals over a three-hour period. The patient is given a 75g drink of glucose solution (Lucozade), which should cause glucose levels to rise in the first hour, and then fall back to normal within three hours as the body produces more insulin to normalize glucose levels.

Blood drawn two hours after drinking the glucose r 7.8 mmol/l is considered normal. Two-hour postload levels of 7.8 mmol/l or higher but less than 11.1 mmol/l are an indication of impaired glucose tolerance. Blood glucose levels of 11.1 mmol/l or higher two-hour postload point to diabetes.

Other Tests

If you are a new patient, your doctor should take a detailed medical history at your initial visit. A thorough head-to-toes physical examination to check for the presence of possible complications of diabetes may also be undertaken. This may include an evaluation of your cardiac (heart) function, blood pressure, and a neurological examination of your reflexes, muscle strength and sensitivity to stimulation.

A monofilament test, which involves touching the bottom of your foot with a piece of fibre resembling a thick strand of fishing line, is an easy and inexpensive way to establish if you have lost sensation in your feet due to nerve damage – a condition called peripheral neuropathy.

Your feet will also be examined carefully for infection, ulceration and circulatory problems. A weak pedal pulse (pulse taken on the foot) is an early sign of peripheral vascular disease, or PVD, a condition where some blood vessels outside of the heart become narrowed or blocked and, as a result, blood flow is reduced to the surrounding tissues – often the hands and feet. For more information on monofilament testing, PVD, neuropathy and other complications of diabetes, see Chapter 15.

Other tests that may be performed at or shortly following your initial diagnosis include:

·   A urine test for microalbumin, a protein that can indicate problems with kidney function
·   An HbA1c blood test, to see what your longer-term three-month blood glucose average is
·   A fasting blood lipid profile, to check cholesterol levels
·   A TSH (thyroid-stimulating hormone) test, to check for thyroid dysfunction, a common risk for people with Type 1 diabetes
·   An electrocardiogram (ECG), to assess cardiac function.

Additional tests and procedures may also be indicated, depending on your specific medical history. Chapter 6 has extensive information on laboratory tests for diabetes and diabetes-related complications.

Your Health Care Team

Routine diabetes care requires input from a number of specially trained health care professionals. You will need to see a doctor – this may be a diabetes specialist (diabetologist) based at the hospital, or it may be a GP with a special interest in diabetes. You will also see a diabetes specialist nurse at the hospital, or a practice nurse with special training in diabetes care at your local surgery. A third, and equally important, member of your immediate team will be a state registered dietician.

Diabetes is a systemic disease that has the potential to affect every part of the body; as a result, there are numerous other health care providers with specialized training in various areas who may become involved in your diabetes care. Your doctor will screen for the development of various long-term complications of diabetes, but may refer you to a specialist for further monitoring or treatment if necessary.

The Diabetes Clinic

Once you have a confirmed diagnosis, you will probably be referred to a diabetes clinic – this may be a small surgery that is held by your GP with the help of a practice nurse, or you may be referred to a larger clinic at your local hospital. The components of diabetes care should be the same, wherever you go.

Communication is Key

So exactly what defines good communication? It's talking with one another rather than at one another – listening instead of just hearing, and explaining rather than commanding. If you ask your doctor why he has ordered a certain test, he should be able to explain it in layperson's terms. And if your doctor has questions about your self-care, you should be forthright and honest so he can provide you with the best care possible.

Here are a few other suggestions you may find useful in improving communication with your doctor, nurse, dietician or health care specialist:

· Think about the symptom(s), questions and treatment issues you want to discuss in advance. Bring notes if necessary.

- Bring your medications (in their original bottles) with you. This should include herbs and supplements – your doctor should know what you're taking because some supplements may interact with other medications or may be inappropriate for diabetes patients.
- Treat your doctor as you would like to be treated yourself – respectfully and candidly.
- Bring someone else along to join you after the examination to hear what the doctor is recommending.
- Take your pills as prescribed, and if you do not, let your doctor know so you can discuss an alternative.
- Don't be a 'DNA (did not attend)' for appointments, and let the receptionist know exactly what you need to see the doctor for so she can book your appointment for an adequate length of time.

Ophthalmologists

The blood vessel damage associated with diabetes puts you at risk for diabetic retinopathy and other vision problems. Ideally, you should see a specialist doctor trained in eye diseases – an ophthalmologist – to treat existing eye disease and to screen for problems. An optometrist (an eye care professional who is not a physician) may also screen for diabetic retinopathy. All people with diabetes should have a dilated eye examination once a year as part of their 'annual review'.

Mental Health Professionals

The psychological toll of diabetes can be a tremendous burden, both emotionally and physically. Up to 20 per cent of people living with diabetes also suffer from depression. Therapists, psychiatrists, psychologists and/or trained counsellors can help you cope with the stresses of diabetes; support groups are also a great resource for coming to grips with diabetes and learning from the experiences of others.

Nephrologists

Because diabetes is the number one cause of chronic kidney disease, you may see a nephrologist – a physician specializing in renal care.

Podiatrists

Proper foot care and regular examinations of the feet are extremely important in diabetes care, so a podiatrist, or foot doctor, is also a key member of the health care team. Podiatrists can detect and treat neuropathy (nerve damage) of the feet and foot ulcers. They can also help educate patients on preventative foot care.

Other Specialists

Other specialists that may be on your diabetes health care team include the following:

- **Gastroenterologist:** A doctor who specializes in diseases and disorders of the digestive tract.
- **Gynaecologist:** A doctor who specializes in women's reproductive medicine.
- **Obstetrician:** A doctor who monitors pregnancy and birth.
- **Urologist:** An doctor with special training in treating the urinary tract.
- **Neurologist:** A specialist of the central nervous system (CNS), who treats CNS disorders as well as those of the peripheral nervous system, such as neuropathy.
- **Dermatologist:** A doctor who treats skin diseases and disorders, and may have special training in wound care.
- **Physical therapist:** A trained health care professional who assists in strength and mobility recovery through exercise and other techniques.

Coordinating Care

There may be a number of different health care providers all having some input into your overall diabetes care and management; it's important that all the team players are communicating effectively with each other and with you. There are some steps that you can take in order to help keep things in line.

- Keep a running list of which specialists you are seeing for what.
- Ask for hard copies of test results whenever possible.
- Keep a running list of all medications prescribed to you, and take this to all of your appointments.
- Take notes of questions, concerns and new issues raised at appointments with doctors and specialists.

Remember, your health care providers work for you, but you are the one ultimately in charge of your own health care. Don't be shy about following up on your treatment, and don't let any doctor or medical staff make you feel guilty about doing so.

Getting a Good Education

Since you spend most of your time away from the doctor's surgery, it's important to learn as much as you can about how you can manage your diabetes and prevent complications at home. In fact, diabetes is such a complex disease that it merits its own course of study. Self-care, a generalized term for looking after yourself and promoting wellness, is the main thrust of diabetes education. You'll also learn essential skills like testing blood glucose levels and injecting insulin.

Your diabetes education will involve the members of your health care team and perhaps your local Diabetes UK voluntary group or support group. In addition, you can learn much about diabetes from books, the Internet and patient information available from your doctor's surgery.

The National Institute of Clinical Excellence (abbreviated to NICE; part of the NHS) has recently issued guidance on patient education for diabetes. It recommended that structured education should be made available to all people with diabetes at the time of diagnosis, and then as required on an ongoing basis based on a formal assessment of need.

Going to School

Group education for people with diabetes is now becoming more widely available. Your diabetes nurse should be able to refer you to any appropriate sessions that are running in your area. Your local Diabetes UK voluntary group may also host education classes.

Diabetes classes cover a wide range of issues, including how diabetes affects your body physically and emotionally, how to test blood glucose levels, the importance of exercise, knowing the signs of a hypo, regulating medications and/or insulin, preventing the development of complications, and coping with lifestyle issues. Of course, one of the main teaching points is about diet and diabetes. Courses may be run by a team of health care providers, each having their own specialist input.

f@ct

> Your diabetes specialist nurse and dietician each have a specific role to play in your education. If you do not automatically get to see these health care professionals at the diabetes clinic, ask your doctor for a referral. Your diabetes nurse will work with you to ensure that what you learn is tailored to your own personal needs and cultural preferences.

Dietary management is one of the cornerstones of diabetes care, especially in Type 2 diabetes, where weight loss may also be an issue. A state registered dietician or a nutritionist who works with patients with diabetes is an essential part of your care team.

Your dietician can teach you concepts like carbohydrate counting and explain how certain foods affect blood glucose levels. Most important, your dietician can also work with you on a one-to-one basis to design a meal plan that fits your particular lifestyle – if you're a vegetarian, it will do you little good to get a fish and meat menu, for example. If you have a job that keeps you out on the road a great deal of the time, you need someone who can help you make healthy choices outside of the kitchen. Working closely with your dietician will enable you to develop menus and meal plans based on reality.

Dose Adjustment For Normal Eating (DAFNE) programs are special education courses for people with Type 1 diabetes, teaching insulin adjustment based on food intake. This approach to diabetes management is particularly suited to young adults who yearn for more 'dietary freedom'.

Taking Control

In diabetes-care lingo, control is maintaining blood glucose levels as close to normal (non-diabetic) levels as much of the time as possible. Diabetes UK recommends that people with diabetes aim for blood glucose levels between 4 and 7 mmol/l before meals and less than 10 mmol/l at two hours after meals.

It is important to remember that the target goals are general recommendations only, and you will work with your doctor to determine the blood glucose goals that are right for you and your particular health picture. If you haven't worked it out already, while there are many guidelines and targets in diabetes care, in practice just about everything about the disease varies by individual. A food that sends one person's blood sugar off the charts may cause barely a ripple for another.

Is your head spinning yet? With all the information thrown at you, both from your health care team, from books and other literature, and from well-meaning friends and relatives (who quite frequently spread misinformation rather than fact), being overwhelmed is completely normal. Take a deep breath and remember three things:

1. You aren't in this alone – your health care team is there to help.
2. You don't have to learn it all at once – control involves some trial and error.
3. Reinventing the wheel is not necessary – others have gone before you, and you'll find getting through the physical and emotional demands much easier if you join a support group and draw on their wisdom.

Frequent blood glucose testing, careful monitoring of what and how much you eat, exercise and other lifestyle adjustments are the paths to achieve control. In some cases, 'power tools', such as oral medications or insulin, may also be necessary.

A Treatment Triad

Treatment for the disease won't be as simple as collecting your prescription and getting back to business as usual. People living with

Type 1 diabetes will rely on insulin as their main weapon against complications, but diet and exercise also play an important role.

Those with Type 2 diabetes may be able to use diet and exercise to effectively keep their blood sugar levels under control. Often, a little help from oral medications or insulin is also required. If you need medication to control your diabetes, that doesn't make you any less successful at managing your disease than someone who has been able to do it through diet and exercise only. Together, diet, exercise and medication are simply different tools designed to help you achieve the same goal – normal blood glucose levels.

Eat Properly

If you have Type 1 diabetes, what you eat determines how much insulin your body requires, so knowing how food choices affect your blood sugar is essential.

Because over 80 per cent of people with Type 2 diabetes are overweight or obese, eating for both blood glucose control and weight loss is often a fundamental component of Type 2 care. Appropriate food choices and dietary considerations for diabetes are covered in detail in Chapter 11.

Exercise

Exercise is fundamental to good health and well-being. It lowers blood glucose levels, improves heart health and promotes weight loss in overweight people with Type 2 diabetes. However, people with diabetes do need to take precautions with their exercise routine to ensure that they don't experience a hypoglycaemic episode. Chapter 12 has further details on getting fit with diabetes.

Medication

While some people are able to successfully manage their Type 2 diabetes through diet and exercise, many others require the additional assistance of oral medications. Turn to Chapter 9 for detailed descriptions of prescription drugs used in Type 2 treatment.

Health care professionals in the UK look to a number of professional guidelines for the diagnosis and management of diabetes; these have been published by Diabetes UK, the National Institute of Clinical Excellence (part of the NHS) and other organizations, including the World Health Organization. See Appendix C for an overview of clinical care recommendations, guidelines and standards.

Chapter 6

Tests, Tests and More Tests: The Annual Review

Diabetes takes its toll on the body in numerous ways, and since much of the damage is happening while you are blissfully unaware, the prevention and/or early detection of complications is very important. That's why all people with diabetes should have an 'Annual Review', where a number of different tests are performed.

The HbA1c Test

In addition to your self-monitoring routine (covered in the next chapter), you'll be donating quite a bit of blood to the testing cause at your doctor's surgery. One of the most important of these tests is the glycosylated haemoglobin test (also called a glycated haemoglobin test, GHB or HbA1c test). The test assesses your long-term, three-month glucose average.

HbA1c is a substance produced when excess glucose attaches itself to haemoglobin (a substance in red blood cells). The higher your percentage of HbA1c, the higher your blood glucose levels have been over the past 90-day period.

It is recommended that a HbA1c test be performed at least twice annually, and up to four times a year for individuals who are undergoing adjustments to treatment or failing to meet treatment goals.

HbA1c can be measured in the lab using different methods; however, these should be standardized against the HbA1c assay used in the DCCT and UKPDS (see below for explanation). This means that results can be meaningfully compared to risk findings published in the medical literature.

Long-Term Control

HbA1c levels are the best measure of how you're doing in the long term. While home monitoring offers you a single snapshot of where your blood glucose is at a particular point in time, a HbA1c test is like a surveillance camera running for three months, day and night, giving you the big picture of your average blood glucose levels.

The Diabetes Control and Complications Trial (DCCT), a landmark clinical study that took place in medical centres across the United States in the early 1990s, demonstrated that people with Type 1 diabetes were 40–75 per cent less likely to develop neuropathy, eye disease and nephropathy (kidney disease) when they kept their HbA1c values at 7.2 per cent (achieved through an 'intensive care' routine of testing four times daily, keeping in close contact with care providers and participating in diabetes education courses). Follow-up studies of DCCT participants also found that tight control of blood glucose reduced the risk of atherosclerosis (as measured by carotid artery wall thickness), a benefit that remained six years after the DCCT concluded.

Similarly, the United Kingdom Prospective Diabetes Study (UKPDS), another large-scale study, found that participants with Type 2 diabetes who kept their HbA1c values below 7 per cent had a 25 per cent reduction in the incidence of these same complications. And for every percentage point decrease in HbA1c achieved, there was a 35 per cent reduction in the risk of complications. Whether you have Type 1 or Type 2 diabetes, the HbA1c is not only a look back at the past three months, but a glimpse into your future risk of complications.

Certain conditions and substances can affect the results of a HbA1c test. Vitamins C and E, opiates and salicylates such as aspirin can influence results of some tests, as can iron deficiency anaemia and chronic alcoholism.

Determining Your Target Goal

People *without* diabetes have an HbA1c of around 5 per cent. It is possible for people with well-controlled diabetes to achieve HbA1c levels in a range very close to normal. The American Diabetes Association (ADA) suggest a < 7 per cent goal, while the American Association of Clinical Endocrinologists recommends a target HbA1c of < 6.5 per cent.

In the UK, the National Institute for Clinical Excellence (NICE) have published guidelines for Type 2 and are in the process of publishing guidelines for Type 1 diabetes. The Type 2 guidelines recommend 6.5–7.5 per cent as ideal targets, with the actual figure depending on individual circumstances. Consultation documents suggest that the targets published for HbA1c in people with Type 1 diabetes will most probably be similar.

HbA1c readings at and soon after diagnosis are usually high because they reflect your blood glucose levels in the period before your diabetes was diagnosed and treatment started – so do not be discouraged if your initial HbA1c tests are higher. Target HbA1c levels are as individual as diabetes itself. Your doctor will look at your medical history, age, lifestyle and other factors, and will work with you to define a custom target goal specific to your needs. It can take some time to get your HbA1c where you want it.

The risk of macrovascular complications (especially heart disease) becomes more significant as HbA1c rises above 6.5 per cent; the risk for microvascular complications (especially eye disease, kidney disease and nerve damage) becomes more significant as HbA1c levels rise above 7.5 per cent. Individual HbA1c targets take into account your risk factors for these complications.

Home HbA1c test kits are now available (manufactured by Metrika), which use a drop of blood from a finger prick, and display a value for percentage HbA1c in eight minutes. The single-use meters are expensive, however, and most health care professionals in the UK still prefer to use standardized laboratory methods to determine HbA1c levels.

Other Glucose Tests

Your provider may do a random blood glucose test to check the accuracy of your self-monitoring and/or your home meter. She may also test your glucose levels if she is making an adjustment to your medication or treatment routine. Results are provided in plasma glucose values.

The Fructosamine Test

This is another test that measures your blood glucose over a period of time (2–3 weeks, as opposed to the 8–12 weeks measured by the HbA1c test). The fructosamine test is a measurement of glycated serum proteins, and may be used as a companion to HbA1c when you want to find out how blood glucose control has responded to treatment changes in a shorter time period.

Urine Glucose Tests

Available as reagent 'dipstick' tests, urinary glucose tests were once the standard method of measuring glucose levels at home for people with diabetes. With the advent of accurate home monitoring systems, urine glucose tests are now usually relegated to the purpose of infrequent screening.

These tests have several drawbacks. First, they are time-delayed – they can't tell you what your blood glucose level is right now, but only several hours later after glucose has filtered into the urine and urine has collected in the bladder and is ready to leave the body. They are also not highly sensitive or specific; a negative urine test can ensure only that your blood glucose levels are below 10mmol/l – well above a 'controlled' range for the majority of people.

Urine glucose tests may be used by patients who can't or won't blood test due to discomfort or other reasons. If you have hypoglycaemic unawareness, or are prone to excessive low blood glucose levels, it is critical that blood monitoring be used instead of urine monitoring, as urine glucose testing cannot detect when the blood glucose is dropping too low.

Lipid Profile

Because cardiovascular disease is the leading cause of death among people with diabetes, an annual fasting lipid profile as part of regular preventative diabetes care is recommended. If you are working with your doctor to control lipid levels through medication or diet, testing may be done more often.

A fasting lipid profile is a blood test that assesses your risk for developing cardiovascular complications by measuring levels of total cholesterol, high-density lipoprotein (HDL or 'good') cholesterol, triglycerides, and low-density lipoprotein (LDL or 'bad') cholesterol.

It is also used to diagnose dyslipidemia, a condition characterized by high triglyceride and low HDL cholesterol levels that is common in Type 2 diabetes and increases the overall risk of heart disease.

Lipid Assessment Levels for Adults with Diabetes*		
	At risk	**High risks**
Serum total cholesterol	≥ 4.8–6.0 mmol/l	> 6.0 mmol/l
Serum LDL cholesterol	3.0–4.0 mmol/l	> 4.0 mmol/l
Serum HDL cholesterol	1.0–1.2 mmol/l	<1.0 mmol/l
Serum triglycerides	1.7–2.2 mmol/l	> 2.2 mmol/l

* International Diabetes Federation guidelines

Medical history, gender, age, ethnicity and even geographic region of origin can impact cholesterol levels. Triglyceride levels can be raised by kidney and liver disease and alcoholism. High serum cholesterol levels can be triggered by poor dietary habits, pancreatitis, hypothyroidism, lipid disorders and certain kidney and liver diseases. High LDL levels put one at an increased risk of coronary artery disease.

More Cardiovascular Tests

As a rule, your diabetes doctor will assess your risk factors for heart disease every year, especially if you are getting on in life and have Type 2 diabetes. Depending on your risk factors, you might be referred to a heart specialist (cardiologist); there are a number of cardiac tests that may then be performed at the hospital.

Electrocardiogram (ECG or EKG)

An ECG measures the electrical impulses put out by the heart and creates a visual representation, or tracing, of them. The test is used to check for irregularities in heart rhythm or rate and to detect signs of coronary artery disease.

For a resting ECG, you will be asked to lie flat on a table while sensor patches (leads) are attached to ten various points on the body. The sensors are attached to wires that transfer your heart's electrical impulses into the ECG unit, where a tracing is generated. The test is very brief, taking only about five to ten minutes from start to finish. Your physician will then review the tracing for abnormalities that may indicate an artery blockage or other heart problems.

Exercise Stress Test

As the name implies, an exercise stress test evaluates how your heart and cardiovascular system perform under the pressure of exercise. Your heart is again monitored with ECG leads and a blood pressure cuff. A pulse oximeter (a small, painless clamp that uses light to measure the level of oxygen in your bloodstream) is attached to a finger or other site with sufficient blood flow. Baseline levels of your heart function are taken at rest before the stress test begins.

A stress test is usually performed on a treadmill or stationary bicycle. The level of exertion, or stress, is increased periodically until the patient reaches a specific heart rate. Each time the stress increases, vital signs are measured. The test will be stopped if chest pain, high blood pressure or other danger signs develop. The whole procedure typically takes about 15–20 minutes, and your heart will continue to be monitored after the exercise portion ends until vital signs return to baseline levels.

Echoes and Scans

Your doctor may also recommend other tests that assess cardiac function and structure, including nuclear perfusion and echocardiography. Nuclear perfusion tests, such as a thallium scan, use a trace amount of radioactive material injected into the bloodstream. The radioactive material is absorbed by cardiac muscle and allows better visualization of the heart structures using a special camera. Poor absorption is associated with inadequate blood flow (perfusion) and may indicate that the arteries leading to that portion of the heart are diseased.

Echocardiography, or 'echo', uses ultrasound to create an image of the heart. A small wand, called a transducer, is passed over the chest and sound waves emitted by the transducer bounce off the structures of the heart. The resulting picture is displayed on a video screen. Blood flow is also visible.

Kidney Function Tests

Diabetes is the leading cause of chronic kidney failure, the end stage of renal disease (ESRD). Uncontrolled high glucose levels can damage the nephrons – the filtering units of the kidney that remove excess fluids and waste products from the bloodstream. Regular screening for early signs of kidney problems is an essential part of diabetes care.

Testing for Protein in the Urine

Healthy kidneys should filter and absorb proteins, not excrete them into the urine. Tests for very small amounts of protein in the urine (microalbuminuria) detect the early signs of kidney damage. Assessing more extensive loss of protein in the urine (proteinuria) is an important part of monitoring the extent of kidney damage.

Tests for protein in the urine are usually carried out at diagnosis and at least annually thereafter. If you have a history of kidney problems or are at high risk for renal disease, these tests may be performed more frequently. Protein in the urine is also tested for during pregnancy.

Chemical reagent test strips (dipsticks) may be used to test for protein in the urine. They are quick and easy, requiring only a small sample and a few minutes at most for testing. However, timed urine collections – over 24 hours, for example – give a more accurate picture of how much protein is being lost by the kidneys.

Detecting low levels of protein (albumin) in the urine is the first sign of kidney damage due to diabetes (diabetic nephropathy). Microalbuminuria relates to the loss of very small amounts of albumin in the urine and is a risk factor for kidney disease and cardiovascular disease as well.

Proteinuria (or macroalbuminuria) relates to a much greater loss of albumin in the urine and represents the progression of kidney disease to the next stage.

You will usually be asked to take an early morning sample with you to your Annual Review appointment for protein testing. If microalbuminuria or proteinuria is present, you will probably have the test repeated twice more within the next month, if possible.

Protein in the urine can also indicate infection and other urinary tract disorders. Bladder infection and/or nephritis can cause some protein to be lost in the urine, as can high blood pressure and extended periods of hyperglycaemia.

Urine Creatinine Clearance

A creatinine clearance test is sometimes performed to assess kidney function. The test measures the kidney's ability to filter creatinine from the blood. Creatinine is a metabolic by-product of creatine, the amino acid that supplies energy for muscle contractions. Normal kidneys should filter creatinine, a waste product, into the urine at a constant rate.

Before a creatinine clearance urine test is performed, a blood sample is taken to determine the level of creatinine in the bloodstream. You are then given a container to collect urine output for 24 hours. The final specimen is analyzed for creatinine output, and the creatinine clearance is computed by comparing the urine creatinine to the original blood creatinine levels. The test gives an indication of glomerular filtration rate (GFR); if kidney function is impaired, creatinine levels will be low.

It is recommended that this test be performed five years after diagnosis in individuals with Type 1 diabetes, immediately following diagnosis in people with Type 2 diabetes, and at least annually thereafter for both Type 1 and Type 2. It may be performed more often with those patients at high risk for renal disease.

Low creatinine clearance levels indicate kidney disease (i.e. polycystic kidney disease, glomerulonephritis, renal cancer), congestive heart failure and/or severe dehydration.

Serum Creatinine

Serum (or blood) levels of creatinine are usually measured at least once per year at the Annual Review. Serum creatinine levels are used in assessing kidney function and used in calculations for the creatinine clearance test. If serum creatinine levels are greater than 150 µmol/l you may be referred to a kidney specialist (nephrologist) for further assessment.

Can't keep your creatinine correct? Just remember that healthy, functioning kidneys will cleanse this waste product from the blood and move it into the urine for disposal – so serum levels should be low and urine levels should be high.

Plasma Urea

Urea is another waste product that is filtered from the blood by the kidneys. Urea is generated in the liver by metabolized protein. Your plasma or blood level can help your doctor determine your glomerular filtration rate (GFR), or the rate at which your kidneys are filtering waste and fluids from your body. Elevated urea levels indicate a slowdown in kidney function. The normal range for plasma urea is 3.0–6.5 mmol/l; higher levels may indicate reduced kidney function.

Dilated Eye Examination

Diabetes can cause blood vessels in the retina to become damaged or blocked, resulting in vision loss – a condition known as diabetic retinopathy. It is estimated that half of all people with diabetes will develop retinopathy at some point in their lifetime. They are also at risk for developing cataracts and glaucoma, which may impair vision.

All people with diabetes should have a dilated eye examination at least once a year. If you have Type 1 diabetes and have no known vision problems, the first examination may be between three and five years following initial diagnosis after the age of ten; for Type 2 diabetes, it should be at or shortly following diagnosis. If you have diagnosed eye disease, you may require more frequent assessment to monitor treatment and disease progression.

In a dilated eye examination, eyedrops are used to counteract the reflexes that normally trigger the pupil to shrink in bright light. The ophthalmologist uses a high-intensity focused light called a slit-lamp to illuminate the eye. Dilation opens up the pupil, allowing the ophthalmologist to view the back, or fundus, of the retina and the blood vessels and optic nerve situated there.

Pregnant women with pre-existing diabetes (not gestational diabetes) should have a dilated-eye examination during the first trimester of pregnancy to check for microvascular (blood vessel) problems. Additional eye examinations may be indicated, depending on your medical history and the outcome of the initial examination.

An intraocular pressure test, also called a tonometry test, is used to check for glaucoma. Tonometry is sometimes called a 'puff test' because it may involve blowing a quick puff of air into your eye and measuring the resistance it meets. Another type of pressure test, applanation, uses fluorescein dye to temporarily colour the cornea before a tonometer instrument is placed against the eye to measure fluid pressure. Anaesthetic drops are used to relieve any discomfort.

Other parts of a comprehensive eye examination may include the following tests:

· **Visual acuity test:** The familiar 'big E' Snellen eye chart
· **Visual field test:** A test of your peripheral (side) vision
· **Refraction test:** This checks your ability to see an object at a specific distance
· **Binocular test:** Assesses your eye teamwork – how well the muscle coordination and control of your eyes work in tandem.

If you wear glasses or contact lenses, your examination should also include an evaluation of your current prescription.

Chapter 7

Self-Monitoring of Blood Glucose

A home blood glucose meter – a device that analyzes a blood sample and gives you a reading of your current blood glucose levels – is the next best thing to having a lab in your medicine cabinet. A meter is probably the single most useful tool you have for knowing what's going on with your diabetes, mainly because it is always accessible, provides instant results, and doesn't require a trip to the surgery.

Why Test?

Regular self-monitoring of blood glucose levels (sometimes abbreviated to SMBG) gives you a quick clinical snapshot of exactly where your blood glucose levels are at any given moment. Testing, and keeping a detailed log of test results and the circumstances that surround them, will help you understand how certain foods and activities affect your blood glucose. Once you are able to detect patterns in blood glucose changes over time, you can use the information to adjust your treatment to suit.

I can't stand the thought of using a needle on myself. Can't I just test for sugar in my urine?
You could, but it would do little to help you control your diabetes. Urine glucose testing was the way it was done before home glucose meters became commonplace. But because urine collects and mixes in your bladder for several hours before it leaves the body and only contains glucose when blood levels are more than about 10 mmol/l, it isn't a very timely or sensitive test. Worse, it cannot help detect potentially dangerous low blood sugar levels.

The Diabetes Control and Complications Trial (DCCT), a landmark clinical study, found that tight control of blood glucose levels using SMBG significantly reduced the risk of diabetes-related complications. Since the study was published in 1993, home testing has become a recommended, routine self-care practice.

Another role of SMBG is to help you assess how effective your medication or insulin is in controlling your glucose levels. It is also an invaluable tool for adjusting the timing of medication to ensure the best possible control.

Perhaps most important, SMBG can help you avoid life-threatening blood glucose emergencies. If you are under stress, ill with the flu or taking medications that affect blood glucose levels, regular testing can help you keep close tabs on your blood glucose levels so you can take action before they go dangerously high.

Testing before, after, and even during exercise can help you avoid a precipitous drop in blood glucose levels. It's also a good idea to test if you've been drinking alcohol, another trigger for hypoglycaemia. If you feel a low coming on, a quick test can confirm your levels so you can take action immediately.

Home glucose blood testing is particularly important for people with a condition known as *hypoglycaemic unawareness*. These individuals have lost the ability to perceive the normal warning signs that blood sugars are dropping too low – such as shakiness, anxiety, sweatiness, hunger, irritability and rapid heartbeat. Without testing, they may lose consciousness before realizing they are experiencing a hypo.

Developing a Testing Schedule

When to test is a matter of debate. Some people test once when they wake up. Others test up to eight times a day – morning, night and before and after meals. As a general rule, when your diagnosis is new and you're learning how different factors affect your diabetes, checking your glucose levels frequently is encouraged. The same holds true for monitoring any changes to your treatment routine.

People with Type 1 diabetes may need to test more than those with Type 2, since they need to use the results to adjust insulin accordingly. People with glucose levels that fluctuate widely, often without warning (a condition sometimes referred to as *brittle diabetes*), may also need to test more frequently than others.

Target Goals

The ultimate goal is to get blood glucose levels as close to normal as possible. However, if you have hypoglycaemic unawareness, or if you have other medical conditions that affect your control, your target glucose levels may be a bit higher. Young children with diabetes who may not yet have the ability to recognize symptoms of hypoglycaemia also tend to have slightly higher goals. You should work with your doctor to establish SMBG goals that are right for you.

The Meter and Other Equipment

Your first order of business is choosing a meter that's accurate, easy to use and comfortable. If you have some latitude in selecting a meter, make sure to ask for recommendations. Your diabetes specialist nurse, members of your support group, and your doctor are all good sources.

Meters are manufactured to be accurate within 20 per cent of laboratory reference values. That may seem like a lot, but as long as your meter is consistent in its readings and you know how much it differs from laboratory values (which your doctor can help you determine), the variance isn't too critical. If a reading seems excessively high or low, try testing again.

Anatomy of a Meter

Blood glucose meters come in all shapes and sizes, but there are some common features that most share:

- **Display.** Blood glucose readings are digitally displayed on a small screen in either whole blood or plasma equivalent results. Both test the amount of glucose in whole blood, but 'plasma equivalent' meters run the results through an extra mathematical formula that displays what the amount of glucose in just the plasma (the fluid in which red and white blood cells are suspended) should be. Because blood glucose tests performed in a laboratory use plasma results, some people find this a convenient feature for comparison purposes. It's important to know what type of numbers your meter is using, since plasma equivalents run approximately 12–15 per cent higher than whole-blood results.
- **Buttons and beepers.** The operator's manual for your meter will explain the button functions. Your meter may also have special audio

signals to let you know when a test is complete, or to alert you to highs and lows.

- **Test strip slot.** Your blood sample goes on a test strip, which is inserted into the meter. Some meters use self-enclosed test strip drums or cartridges, which are automatically fed into the meter and don't require any user handling.
- **Memory.** Most modern meters have some type of memory feature that can record a predetermined number of glucose readings. Some will also let you mark readings taken around insulin doses and generate different average glucose readings.
- **Battery.** Meters are battery-powered, and many have a warning system that will tell you when the battery power starts to get low.

Other features you may find on your glucose meter include large displays or voice modules for patients with vision problems, backlit displays or glow-in-the-dark cases for easy night testing, and computer compatibility for downloading glucose data to special software programs.

tips

Bring your blood glucose meter along to your doctor's appointments. If you're new to testing, or you're using a new brand of meter, your doctor or diabetes specialist nurse can compare the readings with laboratory values to ensure accuracy. In addition, your doctor or nurse may also want to see your technique when you review your self-management.

There are a growing number of meters coming on the market that do more than just test blood glucose levels. The InDuo (LifeScan/Novo Nordisk) is a glucose monitor and an insulin delivery system. The MediSense Optium meter tests both blood glucose and blood ketone levels. The BD Latitude (recently introduced on the US market) is an integrated meter, insulin pen case and supply organizer. These multitasking meters may be a good choice for you if you have Type 1 diabetes and want to cut down on your clutter.

Obtaining the Blood Sample

You draw the blood for testing with a lancet, which is a small, fine needle. Lancets come in a small plastic casing and can be used alone or inserted into a spring-loaded lancing device, which quickly pierces the skin at a preset depth.

Lancets are available in different gauges (such as 21 gauge, 30 gauge). The higher the gauge, the narrower the lancet, and the smaller the insertion hole at the test site. A higher-gauge lancet will, in theory, make for a less painful prick (although factors such as skin sensitivity and test site come in, too). High-gauge lancets may also be preferable for children.

Many meters come with a separate lancing pen, while others have a lancing device integrated into the meter itself. Lancing devices can also be purchased separately. Because each use damages the needle slightly and makes subsequent tests more painful, it's recommended that a fresh lancet be loaded with each test.

The lancets you use depend on three factors:

1. The requirements of the meter
2. The sensitivity and condition of your fingers (for instance, calloused fingers may require thicker lancets)
3. The size of the blood sample required – some meters require a blood drop only as small as a pinhead.

Needlestick injuries are a serious concern, occurring more often than is necessary, from improperly discarded syringes, needles and lancets. You have a responsibility to dispose of such 'sharps' properly. Lancets need to be disposed of in a puncture-proof container, preferably a sharps bin (these bins are available on prescription in England and Wales). Ask at your local doctor's surgery what the procedure is for the disposal of filled sharps containers.

Alternative Site Testing

To the relief of sore fingers everywhere, there is a newer breed of glucose monitors available that allow testing on less sensitive parts of the body, such as the forearm or thigh. These alternative site meters may be a good choice for you if you have sensitive fingers and you find yourself testing infrequently because of it.

However, be aware that test results from alternative sites of the body can vary from fingertip testing. Blood from the fingertips may register glucose changes in the body faster than blood from other testing sites. If you are experiencing signs of hypoglycaemia, or if you have hypoglycaemic unawareness, always test from your fingertips to ensure the most accurate readings.

Test Strips

A test strip is a small rectangular piece of chemically treated paper that collects your blood sample for analysis by your meter. The accuracy of your blood tests depends on the quality and treatment of your test strips, so don't gamble with your health by cutting corners. Using expired strips is dangerous, because they may not be able to detect your glucose levels accurately.

Always keep your test strips out of excessive heat and moisture. The bathroom is a poor choice for storage, as humidity can affect strip accuracy. Storing your strips inside your meter case in their original package will ensure that they stay clean.

Extreme temperature swings can affect the accuracy of meters and test strips. For this reason, avoid stowing your meter and supplies away in your car in hot or cold weather, and don't leave your equipment outside in direct sunlight or extreme cold.

How it Works

So how do you test? First, read the instructions. Even if you're a 'do first, ask for directions later' kind of a person, stifle that instinct. Every meter operates a little differently, and there may be calibration or other steps required that are outlined in the directions for use.

Glucose testing involves using a lancet to prick your fingertip or other area of your body to get a blood sample. When performed on the finger, this is called a finger prick. The blood drop that comes out of the finger prick is then placed on a test strip that has been inserted into the glucose meter. (Many newer meters feature strips that actually draw in or absorb the blood sample.) Once the meter detects an adequate sample of blood on the strip, it will measure the amount of glucose present and display the results on the screen in a mmol/l reading. Some meters will display readings that are excessively high or low with special alarms or warnings. Getting results can take anywhere from a few seconds to a minute.

Following are some tips to improve the ease, accuracy and usefulness of your testing:

- Wash and rinse your hands thoroughly. Any food, medication residue or other substances on your fingers can affect test results.
- Experiment with different gauges of lancets. The thickness, or gauge, of your lancet affects both the size of the blood sample and how painful it feels.
- Experiment with different lancet depths. Spring-loaded lancing devices often offer an option for adjusting how far into the skin the needle pierces.
- Get the blood flowing to your hands before you test yourself. If you have problems getting an adequate drop of blood, running your hands under warm water, rubbing them together or shaking them by your sides can stimulate circulation.

Always have a blood glucose meter close to hand. Having several meters stored at the places where you spend most of your time – home, the office, school or college – will ensure that you can always test if an unexpected high or low hits. If you think you are experiencing a hypoglycaemic episode but don't have a meter with you, take some fast-acting carbohydrates to bring your glucose levels back up, then test as soon as possible.

Troubleshooting

Even with the most fastidious testing methods, sometimes the numbers just won't seem right. If you think your technique may be to blame, review the operator's manual and run the test again. Certain medical conditions (such as anaemia) and substances (such as vitamin C) can influence glucose testing results. Talk with your doctor if you have coexisting medical conditions or are taking medications or supplements other than your diabetes drugs.

Quality Control

If your readings are off, you may be able to use quality-control tools that are part of your meter kit. Control solution is a glucose-based liquid that is used in place of blood to ensure that your meter is working correctly. If the reading on your meter matches the range of values on the control solution label, your meter should be accurate. A special electronic control strip may also be included with the meter; this is used to ensure that it is operating properly. Read your meter instructions to find out more on how to use these features.

Calibration

Glucose monitors must be calibrated for use with your test strips before use. Test strips will be labelled with a number that must be entered into the meter. Check both your owner's manual and test strip documentation for information on calibrating test strip type. If your strips are calibrated correctly and the readings still seem to be off, try one from a new package (and report problems with the old package to the strip manufacturer).

Keep it Clean

A dirty meter or dirty, damaged test strips can give false readings. The instructions for use that came with your glucose meter should tell you how and when to clean it. Be aware that some meters are not designed to be cleaned, so always read the directions first.

Wear and Tear

Even the most rugged meters will wear out eventually. If you're getting frequent error codes or your monitor is giving erratic readings, it may just be time to trade in your trusty old friend for a newer model.

Logging Your Test Results

Your test results are most useful if you view them in the context of the rest of your day. Log your readings, along with your medications, insulin, food intake, exercise and other significant events. Over a period of time, patterns will emerge, and you will probably discover certain triggers that make your blood glucose levels fluctuate. Your doctor can help you interpret the data even further.

Some glucose meters have memory features that allow you to store several weeks' or even months' worth of readings, compute averages, and even indicate which readings occurred in conjunction with a particular insulin dose. These can also be helpful in detecting patterns.

tips

If a reading seems wrong, test again. If it still looks wrong and you feel as if your blood glucose is low, take a fast-acting carbohydrate until symptoms subside. When you're feeling better, call the customer service department of your meter manufacturer and run through any additional troubleshooting steps they offer.

Logbooks

Many meters come with a logbook for recording the results, but a notebook will do the job just as well. When recording your readings, make sure you note the time of the test (i.e. preprandial/postprandial) and the time and amount of medication and/or insulin taken. For an even more complete picture of what's happening with your blood glucose levels, you can also note what you eat at each meal.

The sample logbook shown overleaf includes entry spaces for 'before meal' (preprandial) and 'after meal' (postprandial) blood glucose results, plus a space to record the amount of carbohydrate consumed at each meal and the accompanying insulin dose or mixed dose (if applicable). There's also a space for bedtime and snack test readings. A comments area is available for notes on special circumstances that may have affected your blood sugar that day, such as exercise, specific foods and illness.

Logbooks come in many configurations, and may also include space for checking oral medication doses, a record of food intake for each meal and detailed information on daily exercise. Try out a few formats until you find one that works well for you.

Companion Software

An increasing number of meter manufacturers are putting out meters with companion software that analyzes glucose readings both for patients and their health care providers. This software can be an excellent tool for charting long-term progress of glucose control, especially if it has the ability to generate printable reports and charts, and to graph trends. You can also purchase third-party software to track and analyze your blood glucose readings.

Another new trend is the advent of blood glucose monitor modules that can be used with personal data assistants (PDAs) or Palm units. These have the added advantage of being integrated into a device that the user is already familiar with and keeps at hand. They can also easily save and analyze data.

Daily Diabetes Log

Week of: _____

Day	Breakfast		Lunch		Dinner		Bedtime		Other/Snack		Comments
---	Pre / Post	Carbs / Insulin	Pre / Post	Carbs / Insulin	Pre / Post	Carbs / Insulin	Pre / Post	Carbs / Insulin	Pre / Post	Carbs / Insulin	Diet, exercise, ketones, illness, stress
Mon		/		/		/		/		/	
Tue		/		/		/		/		/	
Wed		/		/		/		/		/	
Thu		/		/		/		/		/	
Fri		/		/		/		/		/	
Sat		/		/		/		/		/	
Sun		/		/		/		/		/	
Avg.											

▲ Always record your glucose readings, along with medication, food intake and other important treatment notes.

Ways to Reduce the 'Ouch' Factor

One of the biggest deterrents to frequent testing is the pain and soreness caused by finger pricks. Recently, the most significant and widely available innovation to help solve that problem is the alternative site meter, which allows the patient to replace finger pricks with blood drawn in less sensitive areas of the body, such as the forearm and thigh. These meters may require smaller blood samples than traditional models, but as previously discussed, the readings they give may vary from fingertip readings.

Trend Testing

At time of writing, there are two non-invasive monitoring devices available that are designed to supplement – but not to replace – regular self-monitoring of blood glucose. These products, the GlucoWatch G2 Biographer and the Medtronic MiniMed CGMS (continuous glucose-monitoring system), are useful for recording and identifying blood glucose trends over time. They also both require calibration with finger prick testing.

The GlucoWatch (made by Cygnus, Inc.) uses a low-frequency electrical current to painlessly draw out and measure glucose through the skin. The device, which displays readings on a watch interface at predetermined intervals, stores up to 8,500 glucose readings for up to 13 hours a day. Results can be downloaded into special software that compiles the data and graphs trends.

fact

The GlucoWatch was found to be highly effective in predicting hypoglycaemic episodes in several clinical studies, which is perhaps one of the biggest benefits of the meter. The G2 allows you to set personal alarm levels for high and low readings, and is approved for use by adults and children aged seven and over.

The Medtronic MiniMed CGMS is an implantable device that measures glucose levels every five minutes for up to three days. It consists of a sensor, which is inserted under the skin by a doctor, and a control module that stores the blood glucose data. The sensor reads glucose levels in cellular (interstitial) fluid. The CGMS does not display glucose readings on the module itself. After you've been on the system for three days, your physician can download the blood glucose data using special software and analyze the results.

On the Horizon

One continuous glucose-monitoring device currently under development by SpectRx measures glucose levels in interstitial fluid (ISF). The SpectRx device uses a laser to create microscopic holes through which the ISF is collected. The ISF is then measured in a sensor patch.

Another product, the Symphony (Sontra Medical Corporation), uses ultrasound to detect glucose levels. Insulin pump manufacturer Animas is also developing an implantable sensor that uses infrared spectroscopy to continuously measure glucose levels, which are then transmitted to a remote receiver. A third monitor still in the prototype stage, the SugarTrac (LifeTrac Systems), employs near-infrared light to measure glucose concentration in the earlobe.

Although these particular meters are being developed in the United States, the technology will soon be incorporated into meters that are available here in the UK. Hopefully, the further exploration of glucose monitoring technologies that reduce patient discomfort will increase testing compliance. In the meantime, if finger pricks have you avoiding your meter, a good alternative site meter can help ease your pain.

Chapter 8

Injecting Insulin

All people with Type 1 diabetes require insulin injections to live, and many Type 2 patients end up needing insulin to control their disease. Before the discovery of insulin in the 1920s, the only way to control Type 1 diabetes was through a near-starvation diet, and patients consequently did not have a very long life span. Today, pen-like devices and electronically programmed pumps can deliver precise doses of the life-saving hormone, and new non-invasive forms of delivering insulin are on the horizon.

How Does Injected Insulin Work?

Injected insulin mimics the action of the hormone produced by the body. Once it is injected under the skin and into the subcutaneous (below the skin) fat layer, it starts stimulating glucose uptake by both skeletal muscle and fat cells, while at the same time signalling the liver to slow or stop glucose production.

The first insulin, isolated by Sir Frederick Banting and Charles Best (with help from J.J.R. Macleod and J.B. Collip), was extracted from the pancreas of a cow. The first few decades of insulin therapy used both bovine (cow) and porcine (pig) derived insulin. Today's insulins are created in the laboratory, cultured from bacteria and yeast with a technology known as *recombinant DNA*.

Manufacturers of animal-derived insulin are starting to phase out their bovine (from cows) and porcine (from pigs) insulins. However, some animal insulins are still available in the UK, including those made by CP Pharmaceuticals and Novo Nordisk.

Insulin Types and Quantities

Insulin comes in several different strengths and actions. A rapid-acting insulin, such as Humalog, is injected immediately before a meal and starts working in under 15 minutes. Its peak of action (when it is working the hardest) is 60–90 minutes after injection, about the time when blood sugar levels would be at their height after a meal. Short-acting insulin starts working 30–60 minutes after injection and peaks in three to five hours. Medium- and long-acting insulins are longer-lasting, with a slower onset and peak action.

Mixtures of shorter- and longer-acting insulins are also available. Pre-mixed insulins are particularly useful for children and the elderly, and in people with vision problems, where drawing up two different insulin types into one syringe might be difficult. Newer long-acting insulins, such as insulin glargine (Lantus), are designed to provide 24-hour coverage.

You and your doctor will choose an appropriate insulin or mix of insulins based on your diabetes and particular blood glucose patterns.

Generalized Classification of Insulins by Type, Onset, Peak and Duration			
Type	Onset	Peak	Duration
Rapid-acting			
insulin analogues			
Insulin lispro (Humalog)	<15 min	30–90 min	<5 hrs
Insulin aspart (Novorapid)	10–20 min	1–3 hrs	3–5 hrs
Short-acting insulins*			
	30–60 min	2–3 hrs	6–8 hrs
Medium- and long-acting insulins*			
	2–4 hrs	6–12 hrs	<24 hrs
			(some last for longer)

*This is a generalized summary of the different kinds of insulins available – each particular insulin has its own specific onset, peak and duration times. For more details on how to find out about specific insulins, see Appendix A.

Insulin Dosage

Your insulin doses will depend on the type(s) of insulin that you use. Your age and lifestyle will both affect whether you stick rigidly to set doses of insulin at the same times every day. Some people may vary their insulin doses according to blood glucose levels, activity levels and diet. Your doctor will advise you on your insulin doses and how/if/when you should vary them.

Selecting the Delivery Device

Insulin must be injected into the subcutaneous layer of fat. At the time of writing, the only approved devices for administering insulin were syringes, insulin pens and air-propelled jet injectors. The type you choose will depend on your insulin prescription, budget and comfort level.

Choosing a Syringe

Syringes are probably the least expensive option, are readily available at virtually any pharmacy, and are easy to operate. If your insulin regime requires mixing two types of insulins that aren't commonly available in a premixed pen, a syringe is your only choice.

Insulin in the UK comes in the standard strength of 100 units per millilitre (called U100), and insulin syringes are specially calibrated and marked for this particular strength. However, in some countries insulin comes as U40 (40 units per ml). If you're travelling abroad, you should be aware of this important difference.

Insulin Pens

Pens are commonly used to give insulin in the UK. They have the benefit of eliminating the step of drawing up insulin from the vial into a conventional syringe. Instead, a pen uses a premeasured insulin cartridge, which usually contains 300 units of insulin. Pens are either disposable, one-use models or reusable. The reusable ones allow you to insert and dispose of insulin cartridges, which come separately. Both types require the use of disposable pen needles, also prescribed separately.

An insulin pen resembles just that, a pen. You uncap it to reveal the pen needle, then 'dial up' your dose by turning the barrel until the correct number of units is displayed. After priming, you put the pen against the injection site, push the needle in and press a button (the plunger) to administer the insulin.

Other Injection Devices

Jet injection devices use air pressure to force insulin through the skin without actually puncturing it. They may cause more bruising than pens and syringes, and can require more training to use effectively. The air pressure must be adjusted to propel the insulin strongly enough to penetrate the skin but lightly enough not to bruise. Finding a balance can take a little time.

For people who are deathly afraid of the needle, a jet injector may be a good choice. Some people find them bulky to carry conveniently, as they are bigger than both syringes and pens.

The only jet injector currently available in the UK is the mhi-500 from The Medical House Plc. The mhi-500 costs £120, but it is available on prescription in England and Wales. Consumables (costing about £6 per month) are also available on prescription.

Injecting Insulin

Before you start, wash your hands thoroughly and examine the bottle of insulin. If you are injecting a clear insulin like lispro, you should look for crystals, cloudiness or debris, and dispose of the bottle if you find any. For users of cloudy, long-acting insulins like Ultralente, gently mix the insulin in the vial by rolling it back and forth between your hands about 20 times. When the colour appears even, it is mixed. Never shake the bottle, as this can damage the insulin. You will also need a syringe (or another device for injecting insulin), and a sharps disposal container.

I'm told I could die if I inject an air bubble along with my insulin!

This refers to air embolism, which can occur when air bubbles are injected into the circulatory system and block a blood vessel (not necessarily fatal). Since insulin is injected into the subcutaneous fat, this isn't a risk. However, bubbles do throw off your dosing.

Drawing up the Insulin

For those of you who use a pen, pump or jet injector, drawing up insulin will not be an issue. Still, it's a good idea to know how to do it in case you are ever without your usual supplies and need to use a syringe. Your diabetes nurse and/or doctor may want to go over this procedure as well.

1. Open the insulin vial or bottle and check the date on the label.
2. Uncap both the plunger and the needle of the syringe.
3. Draw in air to the syringe by pulling out the plunger until the stopper reaches the unit mark of what your insulin dose will be.
4. Push the syringe needle down through the rubber stopper in the insulin vial. Do *not* press down the plunger yet.
5. After the needle is all the way in, push the plunger all the way down to inject the air into the bottle.
6. Turn the syringe and bottle upside down. Make sure that the tip of the needle is still submerged in the insulin. If it isn't, pull the syringe out slightly until it is.
7. Slowly pull the syringe plunger out to draw the insulin until the stopper reaches the correct dosage mark.
8. Check for air bubbles. If there are some, push the insulin back in and redraw until none are visible.
9. Turn the bottle and syringe right-side up and carefully remove the syringe from the vial.

Choosing and Preparing a Site

Insulin should be injected into fat to do its job properly. This makes the fatty areas of the body – the buttocks, abdomen, thighs and back of the upper arms – the most appropriate spots for giving injections. Don't choose your bicep, calf or any other muscular area of your body. Muscle will accelerate the speed of your insulin action, and it hurts more too.

You can't inject yourself in the same spot every time. If you do, lumpy deposits of fat (lipohypertrophy) will form at the site and make injections increasingly difficult. These deposits also slow absorption of the insulin. Injection rotation doesn't require you to move from one side of the body to the other; moving over an inch or so will do the trick. However, you do need to have a method of keeping track of your rotation schedule.

Giving the Injection

Now the moment you've been waiting for – actually injecting the insulin. If you're like most people, you approach the first solo shot with trepidation and possibly fear. Know that you can, and will, do it. Even the most squeamish, needle-fearing patients find that a little practice has them shoving in the syringe without a second thought.

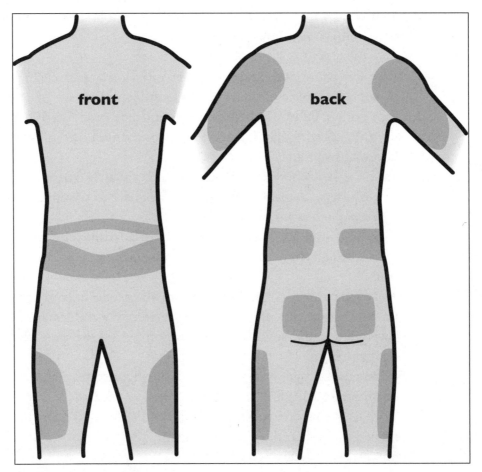

front **back**

▲ GOOD INJECTION SITES

As for giving an injection with an insulin pen, the process is pretty much point and shoot after dialling up the dose. You will need to replace insulin cartridges and needles if you use a reusable pen. Disposable pens come with everything attached. Always read the manufacturer's directions completely for any procedures specific to the model or brand you use.

Your diabetes nurse or doctor will teach you the proper method of finding a good injection site and giving yourself a dose. In fact, you may be given a syringe of saline in the surgery to 'practise' your technique with. After you've chosen an appropriate site, follow these simple steps for giving yourself an almost painless syringe injection:

1. Make sure your hands and the chosen injection site are clean before you start. Be careful not to touch the sterile needle.
2. Grab a roll of fat (or flesh) between your thumb and forefinger with your non-injecting hand. You do *not* want to inject into muscle, so choose appropriately.
3. Assess the area where you're injecting. If it's a fairly fatty site, you can use a 90-degree angle. Otherwise, you may have to try up to a 45-degree angle to avoid hitting muscle or blood vessels.
4. Hold the syringe like a dart, paper plane or anything else you'd want to sail through the air. Keep your thumb off the plunger until it's in.
5. The key to pain-free injection is to stick the needle in completely and quickly. One caution: if you're giving insulin to a child, start a little slower. It may take some experimentation to find the speed that is least painful.
6. Depress the plunger with your thumb slowly and steadily. As you get accustomed to the 'feel', adjust your speed as needed.
7. Count to five before withdrawing the needle slowly. Release the pinched-up flesh and, if necessary, gently press against the site with a clean piece of tissue or cotton wool.

Oral, transdermal (patch) and inhaled insulin may one day be pain-free treatment options. Oral insulin, which is delivered in a spray, has shown the most promise of the three technologies in clinical trials, as the lining of the mouth best absorbs the insulin.

Storing and Transporting Insulin

Hot or very cold cars, bags on the beach and other extreme conditions can quickly deplete insulin's potency. If you're going to be travelling or participating in a recreational activity that will expose your insulin to the elements, make sure you have an insulated case that can keep it safe.

Some insulin manufacturers recommend refrigerated storage of their products; others can be stored at room temperature. Always read the insulin labelling and/or manufacturer's directions for use to find out exactly what storage requirements your particular insulin has.

When Good Insulin Goes Bad

You can tell a lot about insulin just by looking at it. Always check the expiration date of your insulin before you draw it up. Then take a moment to inspect the bottle. Rapid- and short-acting insulin should be clear, while intermediate- and long-acting insulin should look cloudy. The exception to the rule is glargine (Lantus), which is long-acting but is also clear. If your insulin has any crystals or debris in it, or looks cloudy when it should be clear, it could be either expired or spoiled. Never take a chance if it looks questionable; when it doubt, throw it out.

Of course, if you purchase insulin in prefilled pens, a visual inspection is impossible. Make sure to check expiration dates and handle and store pens properly, and you shouldn't have any issues.

Once you open a vial of insulin, its days are numbered, no matter what its expiration date. In general, open insulin has a 30-day shelf life. Always read the manufacturer's directions for use to find out how long a particular type of insulin will last after it has been opened.

All About Insulin Pumps

An insulin pump is a small external device about the size of a pager or cassette tape that is programmed to deliver a slow, continuous infusion (basal dose) of short-acting insulin into the body. At meal times, the wearer programmes a bolus dose to cover the carbohydrates in the food she is going to eat.

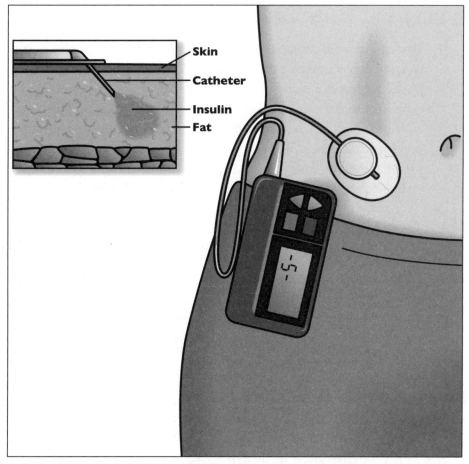

▲ An insulin pump administers insulin through a catheter in the abdominal fat to help control blood glucose levels.

The pump itself consists of a reservoir for holding insulin, a digital display with dose and time information, and a port where the insulin leaves the unit. A piece of plastic tubing called an infusion set hooks on to the pump and carries the insulin from the unit to the body. A flexible plastic cannula or a needle is inserted just under the skin to deliver the insulin. Infusion sets must be changed every two to three days, and insertion sites rotated. Most people use the abdomen for insertion, although the same sites that can be used for insulin injection with a syringe can also be used for insertion.

What are basal and bolus doses?
A basal dose is a slow, continuous infusion of small amounts of insulin that is designed to mimic the insulin secretion of a healthy pancreas. A bolus is a bigger dose of insulin taken before a meal to cover the resulting rise in blood glucose levels. Basal dosing should not be confused with basal insulin (i.e. Lantus), which is taken in a single dose but has continuous, 24-hour non-peaking action.

Who Pumps?

Children who crave added flexibility may be helped by a pump. People with 'brittle' diabetes may find the pump helpful as well, because they can't get a handle on large glucose swings. People who suffer from night-time lows (and accompanying morning highs) may also find that the pump helps them improve control; pumps can be programmed to increase their basal dose as morning glucose levels start to rise (i.e. the dawn phenomenon).

An insulin pump requires a dedicated patient – or, in the case of a small child, a dedicated parent. It is not a 'plug in and play' solution to your diabetes. Blood glucose levels must still be tested at least four times daily, bolus doses for meals have to be computed and programmed, and infusion sets have to be changed regularly. But people who are willing and able to put in the effort often find that the pump gives them that elusive control that injections couldn't.

Practical Matters

Of course, being hooked up to a pump 24/7 brings up all sorts of daily dilemmas. Following are a few pointers on pumps that may answer the more practical questions you may be asking yourself about pump therapy:

- *Many pumps are waterproof, or at the very least water-resistant.* So if you accidentally get them wet, you're covered. There are also a variety of special waterproof and shock-resistant cases available.
- *Infusion sets come with tubing that is more than a metre in length.* The extra length, which doesn't have to be used, comes in handy if you like to put your pump next to your bed at night, or even leave it out of the bath while you bathe or shower.
- *Pumps are worn to bed.* Pumps keep working even when you're sleeping. Good places for your pump to stay at night are under the pillow, in a pyjama pocket or on the nightstand.
- *Pumps can be discreet.* If you don't feel comfortable wearing your pump like a beeper, there are many alternatives. Special pouches and straps are also available to wear pumps on the body under clothing.
- *Pumps can be disconnected, usually for up to an hour.* If you prefer to shower, swim or have sex without the constant companionship of your pump, you can. Always check your blood glucose levels when you hook up again.

Be sure to read the directions for use for your particular pump thoroughly to find out its full range of capabilities. Your doctor, nurse or pump trainer may also have special instructions regarding pump disconnection and other issues.

Pump Therapy in the UK

Only about 0.2 per cent of people with Type 1 diabetes in the UK use insulin pumps – that's compared with about 8 per cent in the USA, 12 per cent in Sweden and 10 per cent in Germany. The main reason for this has been a lack of backing from the health care profession in general, arising from initial problems with pumps in the late 1970s and early 1980s, which led to concerns over their safety. Compounding this has been the lack of experience that the health care providers have had in pump use.

However, insulin pump therapy is available in the UK – there are a number of centres around the country with diabetes health professionals specially trained in pump therapy. If you fit certain criteria, you may qualify for NHS funding for your pump and ongoing consumables. Otherwise, you may have to fork out for it yourself – this might set you back £2,000, plus another £1,000 per year for supplies and maintenance.

If you think that pump therapy might be for you, talk to your diabetes doctor about it. Also contact the pump companies for information; they should be able to provide training for your health care team, as well as for you.

Sharps Disposal

Insulin treatment with any form of sharps produces a lot of medical waste over time. It's important to dispose of needles and lancets properly, to prevent injury to other people in your household and to anyone who comes in contact with your rubbish after it leaves the house.

Special sharps bins are available on prescription in England and Wales. You should collect all used lancets, needles and syringes in them. You may then be required to return the filled sharps bin – ask what the procedure is at your local surgery or pharmacy.

If you don't have access to a sharps return programme, there are many household products that come in containers ideal for sharps disposal. The main requirements are a puncture-resistant, opaque, unbreakable material and an opening that can be easily and tightly sealed.

Label your sharps container 'Used Medical Sharps – Do Not Recycle' with a waterproof marker so everyone who comes in contact with it will handle it appropriately.

When you go on holiday, purchase a compact sharps disposal container for the trip. Another alternative is to use a small puncture-proof case, such as a pencil box or an old thermos, until you return home and can dispose of sharps properly.

Never try to bend or recap a needle or lancet after you've used it. Needle clippers (BD Safe Clip, made by Becton Dickinson) are also available on prescription, and can be used to cut off the needles from syringes and disposable insulin pens. Never try to cut a needle with scissors or a knife. Instead, put your sharps directly into your disposal container.

Chapter 9

Type 2 Oral Medications

If you have Type 2 diabetes, you may not need to rely on regular insulin injections, but there are times when, despite all your best efforts and strict adherence to diet and regular exercise, your blood glucose levels just won't stay down. When diet and exercise fail to do the job adequately, oral medication is the next step. According to results from the United Kingdom Prospective Diabetes Study (UKPDS), three years after diagnosis half of all diet-failing patients will require more than one glucose-lowering therapy.

The Basics

If you are having trouble managing your Type 2 diabetes with diet and exercise alone, your doctor may prescribe an oral medication to improve your blood glucose control. Some people with Type 2 diabetes may also require insulin at some point, but oral medications are almost always given an adequate trial before moving on to insulin. Sometimes insulin therapy will be combined with an oral medication.

There are five main classes of oral medications for Type 2 diabetes: sulphonylureas, biguanides, thiazolidinediones (also called TZDs or glitizones), alpha-glucosidase inhibitors and meglitinides. Combination drugs, which combine medications across two classes of drugs, are also prescribed. Diabetes drugs that are currently on the market work in one of several ways:

· Inhibiting glucose production (biguanides, TZDs)
· Increasing insulin sensitivity (TZDs, some sulphonylureas)
· Stimulating insulin production (sulphonylureas, meglitinides)
· Blocking or slowing the digestion of carbohydrates (alpha-glucosidase inhibitors)
· A combination of two or more of the above actions (the combination drugs).

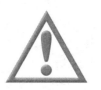

Make sure that your doctor is aware of all other medications – prescription, over-the-counter or herbal – that you are taking. The therapeutic action of your diabetes drug may be affected when taken with certain substances and medicines.

A Smooth Start

When you start on a new medication, log both the amount and timing of the dosage in your blood glucose logbook. This will give you and your health care provider a good idea of the impact the drug is having, and will allow her to make any necessary adjustments. You should note any side effects you have from the drug as well. Side effects will often wane and even disappear completely as your body becomes accustomed to the medication. In some cases, however, a dosage or medication change may eventually be required.

Your doctor should explain both the amount and frequency of your dose and any specific instructions about when to take it. However, it's also a good idea to read the drug labelling and directions for use that your pharmacist provides to ensure that you're taking your medication at the appropriate time and dosage. If the printed instructions seem to vary from what you have been told, call your physician immediately for instructions.

Practical Matters

Medication won't work if you forget to take it, so put your medicines in a place where they are in sight and on your mind. If you take several prescription drugs, a medication organizer may be a good investment for you. There are many on the market, ranging from simple plastic caddies to more elaborate electronic systems. A watch with an audible alarm can also help keep you on track. Some people find keeping their medication with their blood glucose testing supplies convenient.

If you're prescribed a drug that must be taken with meals, keep it on the kitchen table or counter. You should also carry several pills in your purse, car or other 'always with you' spot for meals on the road. Make sure you rotate your extras weekly so they don't expire.

tips

People who take medication to treat their diabetes (either tablets or insulin) are entitled to free NHS prescriptions. Application forms for exemption certificates (which last for five years) are available from your local doctor's surgery or post office (Form FP92A).

Keeping medication within arm's reach can be hazardous in households with small children. Try keeping an empty pill bottle on the table as your reminder, and stow away the full bottle in a childproof cabinet.

Finally, always avoid storing your medications in heat, humidity or direct sunlight, as temperature extremes can cause some drugs to lose their potency. And never take a drug that is past its expiration date.

Sulphonylureas

Sulphonylureas are the oldest class of oral diabetes medication, introduced in the 1950s. There are a number of different types of these drugs available in the UK; some are manufactured by more than one pharmaceutical company, so may be marketed as different brand names. The most commonly prescribed sulphonylureas are glibenclamide (Daonil, Euglucon), gliclazide (Diamicron, Minodiab) and glimepiride (Amaryl). Other less commonly used ones include glipizide (Glibenese), gliquidone (Glurenorm), tolazamide (Tolanase), tolbutamide (Rastinon) and chlorpropamide (Diabinese).

A sulphonylurea may be the first choice of drug for you if you are not overweight, or if metformin is not suitable for you. The oldest of these sulphonylurea drugs – chlorpropamide and tolbutamide – have a relatively low potency, and large doses are required. The newer, or second-generation, sulphonylureas are much more potent and are typically prescribed at much lower doses. These drugs are mostly taken once daily in a single dose, but sometimes they are prescribed in divided doses. Your doctor will tell you when and how often to take your medication. Whatever the schedule, you should always try to take it consistently at the same time from day to day.

How They Work

Called 'hypoglycaemic agents', sulphonylurea drugs work by causing the pancreas to release more insulin, which in turn lowers blood glucose levels. For this reason, sulphonylureas may not be effective in people with long-standing diabetes who have lost most pancreatic beta cell function. Amaryl (glimepiride), the newest of the sulphonylurea drugs, also works to decrease insulin resistance by binding with insulin receptors. So in addition to increasing insulin output, this drug allows the body to more effectively use the insulin it produces.

Possible Side Effects

The most serious potential side effect of the sulphonylurea drugs is a hypoglycaemic reaction, or low blood glucose episode. Significant hypoglycaemia is most commonly a problem with glibenclamide, especially in elderly people and those with kidney problems.

Other possible side effects include, but are not limited to the following:

· Nausea
· Rash and/or itching
· Photosensitivity (sensitivity to sunlight)
· Dizziness
· Drowsiness
· Headache
· Weight gain.

The potential for weight gain can be a problem for overweight patients, as weight gain will work against the benefits of the drug by increasing insulin resistance. Your doctor may prefer to use a newer class of drugs, such as biguanides, for your treatment if you are significantly overweight.

Sulphonylureas (particularly chlorpropamide) also have the potential to react with alcohol, causing nausea, vomiting and facial flushing. Talk to your doctor about this side effect before starting your prescription.

Biguanides

In the UK, metformin (Glucophage, Glucamet, Orabet) is normally the first line of treatment for people with Type 2 diabetes. Biguanides are often preferred over sulphonylureas because they don't cause hypoglycaemia; nor do they promote weight gain. They have also been shown to have a positive effect on blood lipid levels.

Metformin is usually taken two to three times daily with meals.

A 2002 study at the Hospital for Sick Children and the University of Toronto in Canada found that treatment with metformin lowered HbA1c levels and decreased the need for insulin in teenagers with Type 1 diabetes who were considered to be in poor control of their diabetes.

How They Work

Metformin works by suppressing the amount of glucose your liver pumps out. It promotes weight loss and an improved cholesterol profile, which can reduce your insulin resistance. The United Kingdom Prospective Diabetes Study (UKPDS), a landmark 20-year clinical study, found that overweight patients treated with metformin experienced a significantly lower mortality rate than those treated with sulphonylurea drugs and had a marked reduction in strokes and heart attacks.

Possible Side Effects

Metformin is not recommended for people with kidney or liver problems due to the risk of lactic acidosis, a rare but potentially fatal build-up of lactic acid in the bloodstream that occurs when the liver and kidneys do not adequately remove lactic acid. Signs of lactic acidosis include weakness, fatigue, dizziness, breathing problems and unexplained muscle and/or stomach pain. If you experience any of these symptoms while taking metformin, seek prompt medical attention.

Biguanides are also not recommended for use in patients with congestive heart failure. Other potential side effects of metformin include:

- Gastrointestinal distress (bloating, wind and diarrhoea)
- Nausea
- Metallic taste in the mouth
- Depletion of vitamin B_{12} levels.

Because up to 30 per cent of patients prescribed metformin experience gastrointestinal discomfort, dosage is generally started quite low and slowly increased.

If you are undergoing any radiographic (X-ray or CT scan) procedure that involves injection of a contrast medium (i.e. dye) that contains iodine, you should stop taking metformin temporarily because of the increased risk of lactic acidosis. Metformin can be started again if kidney function is normal when it is reassessed 48 hours after the injection.

Thiazolidinediones (TZDs)

Thiazolidinediones, or TZDs, also known as PPAR-gamma agonists, are commonly referred to simply as 'glitazones'. Pioglitazone (Actos) and rosiglitazone (Avandia) are the two TZD drugs currently available in the UK. The first drug in the class, troglitazone (Rezulin), was withdrawn from the market in 2000 after reports of fatalities due to liver damage.

In the UK, the glitazones are licensed for use in combination with either metformin or a sulphonylurea. Actos is usually taken once daily, and Avandia may be taken once or twice daily. Both can be taken with or without food.

If you take birth control pills, TZD drugs can make them less effective. They can also increase fertility in women with polycystic ovary disease (PCOS). Women who take TZD drugs should consult their doctor about contraceptive options.

How They Work

The TZD drugs, which are also called glitazones or insulin sensitizers, target the insulin receptors in muscle and fat cells to increase the level of insulin sensitivity in the body. They also reduce glucose production slightly, and can be effective in lowering blood pressure and triglyceride levels, and in increasing HDL (or 'good') cholesterol. Because they lower glucose so effectively, they also reduce hyperinsulinaemia (excess circulating insulin).

Possible Side Effects

Because of the associations found between Rezulin and liver failure, the National Institute for Clinical Excellence (NICE) stands by the manufacturers' recommendations that liver function be closely monitored in patients taking glitazones. If you take a glitazone, you must have regular testing of the liver enzyme ALT. ALT levels should be tested before treatment starts, every two months for the first year you take the drug, and as recommended by your doctor thereafter. Avandia or Actos should be discontinued if ALT levels rise more than three times the normal upper limit, and should not be started in patients who have ALT levels that are greater than 2.5 times higher than the normal upper limit.

Other side effects of glitazone therapy may include:

· Oedema (water retention) of the ankles or legs
· Anaemia
· Weight gain
· Muscle weakness
· Headaches
· Fatigue
· Cold-like symptoms.

If a blood sugar low occurs when Glyset or Precose is taken in conjunction with a sulphonylurea or insulin, it should *not* be treated with fructose or sucrose (since alpha-glucosidase inhibitors cause a slower digestion of these sugars). Instead, glucose gel or tablets, or milk (which contains lactose) should be used to boost blood glucose levels.

Alpha-Glucosidase (AG) Inhibitors

Acarbose (Glucobay) is the only drug of this type available in the UK. Also called a 'starch blocker', acarbose must be taken at each meal with the first bit of food in order to be effective. Acarbose may be prescribed alongside another glucose-lowering drug as a combination therapy.

How They Work

Acarbose works by slowing digestion. More specifically, it blocks the enzymes responsible for the breakdown of carbohydrates in the intestine, so blood glucose rise is slower and steadier. It may be prescribed for you if you have a hard time keeping your postprandial (after meal) blood glucose levels under control. AG inhibitors may be a preferred therapy in overweight patients, since they do not promote weight gain as the sulphonylureas and glitazones do.

Possible Side Effects

Because of the way they work, most of the side effects of the AG inhibitors are gastrointestinal, and include bloating, diarrhoea, wind and cramp. However, as with metformin, the uncomfortable side effects can be greatly reduced by starting with a small dose and gradually increasing it.

People with serious gastrointestinal disorders, including intestinal disease or obstructions, inflammatory bowel disease and colonic ulceration, should not take AG inhibitors.

If you take oral medications for your Type 2 diabetes and want to become pregnant, make an appointment to discuss your options with your doctor. None of the currently available oral medications are considered safe for use in pregnancy, but insulin is. Your doctor will probably suggest a switch to insulin before you start trying to conceive, so you can stabilize your blood glucose levels on the new therapy.

Meglitinides

Repaglinide (NovoNorm) and nateglinide (Starlix) are currently the only approved meglitinide class drugs in the UK. As with AG inhibitors, they are taken at meal times (usually about 15 minutes before eating) to prevent a postprandial blood sugar rise. People who tend to test high after meals may benefit from treatment with meglitinide drugs.

The meglitinides are sometimes classified as insulin secretagogues, along with sulphonylureas. Repaglinide and nateglinide are rapid-acting compared to sulphonylureas, and may be the preferred choice for tight postprandial control for people who do not have a strict daily routine.

How They Work

Meglitinides are short-acting oral hypoglycaemic agents that bind to and stimulate the insulin-producing beta cells of the pancreas in response to the level of glucose in the bloodstream.

Taken before a meal, meglitinides can boost what is known as *first-phase insulin release*, the production of insulin that is a response to the initial boost of carbohydrate-generated blood glucose after a meal. Both Prandin and Starlix can be taken anywhere from immediately before to up to 30 minutes prior to a meal.

If I miss a meal, should I still take my medications?
First of all, try not to miss meals, as it's hard on blood glucose control. That said, it depends on the type of medication you take and the schedule you take it on. If you take an inhibitor or a meglitinide, you should miss the dose and take the next one with your next meal. As always, talk to your doctor about your specific situation.

Possible Side Effects

Hypoglycaemia can occur as a side effect of the meglitinide drugs. Symptoms of a low blood glucose episode include sweating, shakiness, dizziness, increased appetite, disorientation, heart palpitations, nausea, fatigue and weakness. A hypo should be treated immediately with a fast-acting carbohydrate.

Patients new to Type 2 medications may also experience weight gain with meglitinides. The most commonly reported side effects occurring with meglitinide drugs are as follows.

· Cold and flu symptoms

- Headache
- Diarrhoea and other gastrointestinal complaints
- Joint and back pain.

If you take a meglitinide drug, you should monitor your blood glucose levels one hour and two hours after eating to ensure your medication is working properly. If blood sugar readings still seem too high, talk to your doctor about adjusting your dose.

Combination Therapy

The national clinical guidelines for Type 2 diabetes, issued by NICE, recommend that glucose-lowering therapies should be prescribed on a trial basis, with outcomes monitored using HbA1c measurements. When HbA1c levels start to rise on a given therapy, the guidelines say that another therapy should be added, rather than substituted. So as time goes by, more drugs may be needed to keep blood glucose levels under control. (Eventually, oral medications may fail to be adequate, and this is when people with Type 2 diabetes need to start on insulin.)

Several studies have shown that some diabetes drugs may have the potential to delay or prevent Type 2 diabetes. Metformin reduced the risk of Type 2 diabetes by 31 per cent in the Diabetes Prevention Program (DPP), acarbose reduced the risk by 32 per cent in the STOP-NIDDM trial, and troglitazone (now withdrawn from the market) reduced the risk by 56 per cent in the TRIPOD study.

No Magic Pill

Prescription drugs are never a substitute for appropriate diet and exercise in the treatment of Type 2 diabetes, and ignoring these other two fundamentals of diabetes management is a recipe for disaster. If and when you start medication, stay on track with your diet and exercise programme. You need all three parts of the equation to manage your diabetes effectively.

On the other side of the coin, sometimes people with Type 2 diabetes are reluctant to start on tablets because they feel like they have failed if they can't achieve blood glucose control with diet and exercise alone. Remember that medication is not a crutch, but just another tool for getting your blood glucose levels under control – your main objective in managing your diabetes. You need to take advantage of every tool at your disposal to build a solid and effective treatment programme.

Chapter 10

Food and Blood Glucose

Whether you're Type 1 or Type 2, the food you eat is going to have a major impact on your blood glucose levels, and therefore on your diabetes control and risk of related complications. Although there is no 'diabetic diet', what you eat and when you eat it will form the cornerstone of your diabetes management plan.

All About Carbohydrates

The body begins to convert carbohydrates almost entirely into glucose shortly after carbohydrate-containing foods are eaten. If you have inadequate or insufficient insulin to help process this glucose into cellular fuel, consuming too many carbohydrates can cause blood glucose to rise to dangerous levels. Without carbohydrate-generated glucose you could not function, yet too much can cause irreparable damage.

All foods that contain starches and/or sugars – including fruits, vegetables, milk, yoghurt, breads, grains, beans and pasta – contain carbohydrate. Virtually the only whole foods that are carbohydrate-free are protein-rich meats, poultry and finned fish (when prepared without additional ingredients such as breading, marinade or pickling) and fats such as cooking oils and butter or margarine.

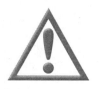

People with gastroparesis, or nerve damage of the stomach, have delayed stomach-emptying issues that causes the normal process of carbohydrate conversion to work differently. If you have gastroparesis or other gastrointestinal/digestive issues, make sure your dietician is aware of them.

To avoid all carbohydrate-containing foods is both impossible and unadvisable – your body needs the important micronutrients and phytochemicals contained in these foods. In fact, the World Health Organization (WHO) recommends that carbohydrates from a variety of foods account for 55 per cent of the total calories in your daily diet. But what you do need to learn is the basics of assessing the quantity and quality of carbohydrates in your food, and how your body reacts to them.

Carbohydrate Science

Carbohydrates are categorized by their chemical structure. A monosaccharide, or simple sugar, is composed of a single saccharide (sugar) chain. Glucose, fructose (fruit sugar) and galactose are all simple sugars. Disaccharides are two simple sugars joined together, and include lactose (milk sugar), maltose (malt sugar) and sucrose (table sugar). Polysaccharides, or complex carbohydrates, are ten or more simple sugar chains joined together. Glycogen, starches and fibre are polysaccharides. (A fourth type of carbohydrate, oligosaccharides, is composed of three to ten sugar chains, but most of these are usually formed from the breakdown of polysaccharides.)

All carbohydrates are broken down into monosaccharides before they can be processed by the body. Amylase, a type of enzyme found in the saliva and secreted by the pancreas, helps to break down carbohydrates into glucose during their journey through the small intestine. Once hydrolysis occurs, the resulting glucose is absorbed into the bloodstream. Any excess is converted to glycogen and stored in the liver.

The Glycaemic Index

Does it matter what kind of carbohydrates you consume? At one time, nutritionists believed that people with diabetes should avoid simple sugars (monosaccharides and disaccharides) and eat foods containing complex carbohydrates instead, with the mistaken belief that simple sugars would raise glucose levels faster and more dramatically across the board. But it's now known that gram for gram, complex carbohydrates found in breads, cereals, potatoes, vegetables and other foods raise the blood sugar approximately the same amount as simple sugars such as honey, fructose or table sugar.

However, there may be a difference in how rapidly certain foods raise blood glucose levels. The glycaemic index, or GI, is a measure of how quickly the carbohydrates in certain foods are transformed into blood glucose. Foods with a low GI (beans, multigrain bread) raise glucose levels at a slower and steadier rate than a high-GI food (rice, potatoes).

The GI of foods does not necessarily correspond to a specific carbohydrate 'type' – some complex carbohydrates may have a higher GI than simple carbohydrates. For people with diabetes, the GI can be an effective tool for avoiding blood glucose spikes.

Carbohydrates and Blood Glucose Control

Carbohydrates and the glucose they generate are an energy source – the dietary fuel of the human body. Insulin produced by the pancreas enables our cells to burn this carbohydrate-generated glucose. This is why determining the amount of carbohydrates in a meal is so important for blood glucose control.

People with Type 1 diabetes, and some with Type 2 diabetes, have to inject enough insulin to accommodate, or 'cover', all the carbohydrates they eat. Many people with Type 2 diabetes have the added task of having to adjust their diets to lose excess weight as well. Concepts like carbohydrate counting and dietary exchanges enable people with diabetes to effectively manage their blood glucose levels.

It's also important to understand that carbohydrates don't work in isolation. Other nutrient components of the food you eat can also affect carbohydrate absorption. High-fat and high-protein foods can delay this absorption. And although fibre is considered a carbohydrate, high-fibre foods also slow the absorption of glucose, since they slow the passage of food through the digestive tract.

Why Fibre is Important

Dietary fibre is often classified according to its solubility in water. Soluble fibre is founds in oats, pulses and citrus fruits. Insoluble fibre (roughage) is mainly cellulose, the major component of plant cell walls. This type of fibre can be found in wheat bran, nuts, grains and vegetables. Soluble fibre is fermented in the gut, producing gases. Insoluble fibre passes through the gastrointestinal system largely undigested, and doesn't contribute significantly to blood glucose levels.

Increased consumption of soluble fibre has been reported to decrease LDL cholesterol levels and may be useful in preventing heart disease. Insoluble fibre may be beneficial in the prevention of constipation, haemorrhoids (piles) and colon cancer. Fibre is an important nutritional tool for helping to normalize blood glucose levels – it slows digestion, and therefore slows the absorption of nutrients (including glucose).

How it Works

When viscous (water-soluble) fibre absorbs water in the gastrointestinal tract, it turns to a gel-like, viscous substance that helps to normalize blood glucose and insulin levels by slowing the passage of food through the intestines. The delay in nutrient absorption means a slower and more stable rise in blood glucose levels.

Because it absorbs the excess intestinal bile acids that help to form cholesterol, soluble fibre has also been shown to help lower blood cholesterol levels, another important consideration in people with diabetes who are at risk of cardiovascular disease.

Another benefit is that viscous fibre improves satiety, or the feeling of fullness you get when eating a fibre-rich meal. It delays stomach emptying, and in those people with Type 2 diabetes who are also overweight, satiety can be a useful tool for weight loss.

Always consume plenty of water or noncaffeinated beverages – at least 2l, or around eight glasses, daily – if you are eating a fibre-rich diet. Fibre without adequate fluids can lead to constipation. Increasing fibre intake slowly can also help to ease any bloating or other unwanted gastrointestinal distress.

Recommended Intake

There are no specific recommendations for a daily fibre intake for people with diabetes in the UK. The main message is to choose high-fibre options wherever possible. The UK Food Standards Agency recommend a daily fibre intake of 20g for men, and 16g for women.

A diet high in low-glycaemic whole-grain cereal fibre has been found to have a beneficial effect in controlling postprandial (after meal) blood glucose levels and reducing serum cholesterol levels in people with Type 2 diabetes. The American Diabetes Association recommends a daily dietary intake of 20–35g of fibre, the same recommended dietary allowances (RDA) as for people without diabetes, to promote good control and cardiovascular health. However, some studies have shown a glucose- and lipid-lowering benefit with fibre intake of up to 50g daily. Talk to your doctor and dietician about what level of fibre in your diet is right for you.

Fibre intake has also been associated with a reduction in diabetes risk in a number of studies. One of these, the six-year Nurses' Health Study, carried out in the USA and involving more than 65,000 participants, found that women on a low-fibre diet heavy in processed, sugary foods were 2.5 times more likely to develop Type 2 diabetes than those who ate at least 25g of fibre daily.

Sugar is Not the Enemy

The no-sugar myth is probably one of the biggest misconceptions about diabetes. The reality is that it isn't sugar specifically that raises blood glucose levels – in reality it's any food that contains carbohydrates, including honey, fruit, milk and vegetables, to name a few. So whether it's a spoonful of sugar, a piece of cake or a banana, it will cause blood glucose levels to rise.

Sugar Alcohols

A sugar alcohol is, quite simply, a monosaccharide that has been chemically transformed into its alcohol form. There are a number of naturally occurring sugar alcohols (also called polyols), including sorbitol, mannitol, xylitol, lactitol, maltitol, isomalt, erythritol and hydrogenated starch hydrolysates. Because they are not completely absorbed in the gastrointestinal tract, the rise in blood glucose levels that they cause is less than with sucrose, which is why people with diabetes may find them desirable. Polyols are frequently used as a sweetener and bulking agent in processed foods marketed as sugar-free.

Because children have a lower tolerance for sugar alcohol sweeteners, check the labels of 'sugar-free' foods carefully and be cautious with the amount of sugar alcohols your child consumes.

In addition, some people find that sugar alcohols have a laxative effect, causing diarrhoea and/or wind.

Artificial Sweeteners

As opposed to naturally derived sugar alcohols, artificial sweeteners are synthetically manufactured sugar substitutes. There are five types of artificial sweetener approved for use in the UK:

- **Aspartame (NutraSweet):** This sweetener is 180 times sweeter than table sugar. Aspartame has been the subject of much controversy regarding potential health effects, but there is currently *no* clinical research that indicates that the sweetener is unsafe for most people (except for individuals with advanced liver disease, pregnant women with hyperphenylalanine or high levels of phenylalanine in the bloodstream, and those with a rare genetic condition known as *phenylketonuria*, or PKU).
- **Saccharine:** The oldest artificial sweetener, saccharine was discovered in 1879 and has been used as a sweetener in foods and beverages for over a century. Saccharine has been linked to bladder cancer in rats, but there is no hard data establishing that normal amounts of the sweetener are dangerous for humans. Saccharine is about 300 times sweeter than table sugar.
- **Acesulfame potassium:** Acesulfame potassium, also called acesulfame K, is 200 times sweeter than table sugar, and studies have confirmed its safe use in people with diabetes, pregnant and nursing women, children and the general population.
- **Sucralose (Splenda):** Sucralose is unique in that it is actually derived from table sugar. However, unlike table sugar it has no carbohydrates, no calories, and it passes through the body almost entirely undigested. The sugar substitute is 600 times sweeter than table sugar. Because it is very stable and withstands temperature changes well, it can be used in cooking and baking. Extensive clinical studies have uncovered no safety risks for people with diabetes and the general population.

- **Cyclamate:** This sweetener is 30–35 times sweeter than table sugar. Cyclamate is often found combined with saccharine (this increases the sweetening power).

If it's sugar-free, does that mean I can eat as much as I want?
Don't be misled by a 'sugar-free' label. Foods containing polyols and/or artificial sweeteners may still contain carbohydrates and calories that should be figured into your meal plan. Read the nutrition facts on the label to get the full story.

Calorie Intake

Ideal calorie intake is based on your activity level, gender, age and other factors. Many people with Type 2 diabetes also face weight-loss challenges; since reducing calorie intake is one component of an effective weight-reduction programme, it is an important consideration in dietary management of diabetes.

According to the UK Food Standards Agency, an average man needs about 2,500 calories a day, and an average woman about 2,000 calories. However, these are generalized figures. Someone who doesn't do much exercise is likely to need fewer calories than a very active person; a tall woman may require more calories than a short man. You should speak to your dietician to determine your own calorie requirements.

It's More Than Just the Calories

If you are overweight and have Type 2 diabetes, keep in mind that even modest weight loss can decrease insulin resistance and improve control. But calorie reduction alone rarely leads to long-term weight control. UK guidelines recommend a comprehensive approach of reduced calorie intake (500 calories less per day), regular exercise, reduced fat intake, education and behaviour modification therapy for long-term success.

The nutrient balance in the food your calories come from is also important. No more than 35 per cent of total calories should come from fat. Carbohydrates and monounsaturated fat together should account for 60–70 per cent of total calories.

Fats and Cholesterol

Fat insulates the body and supplies energy when no carbohydrate sources are available. It also enables the body to absorb and process the fat-soluble vitamins A, D, E and K. However, too much saturated fat and cholesterol can increase the risk of atherosclerosis and other cardiovascular complications from diabetes.

The dietary supplement chromium picolinate has demonstrated an insulin-enhancing effect in several clinical studies, though most available information suggests that it does not help in reducing elevated glucose levels in Type 2 diabetes. Before taking any supplement, always consult your doctor.

All Fats Are Not Created Equal

Fats are confusing to many people when they first start learning the ropes about dietary management of diabetes. The off-target message that all fat is bad has entrenched itself in popular dietary culture; fat-free food production is now a multimillion-pound industry. While some fats are bad for you in excess, others can actually help improve your cholesterol profile. Here are the basics on dietary fats:

- **Saturated fat:** Solid fats that are found in meat and dairy products and vegetable oils. They are associated with high LDL (bad) cholesterol levels.
- **Unsaturated fat:** Either polyunsaturated (e.g. safflower oil) or monounsaturated (e.g. olive oil). Fish and seafood are good sources of unsaturated fat. These types of fats (polyunsaturated in particular) have been shown to be effective in reducing total and LDL (bad) cholesterol levels.

- **Transfats/hydrogenated fats:** Transunsaturated fatty acids, or unsaturated liquid fats that have been processed into a more saturated and solid form by adding hydrogen. They are often found in processed baked goods and commercial fried foods, and may be called 'partially hydrogenated' or 'hydrogenated' fats. Transfatty acids can raise LDL (bad) cholesterol and lower HDL (good) cholesterol, and their use should be limited.
- **Essential fatty acids:** Fish and fish oils and certain seeds and nuts and their oils (e.g. flaxseed, vegetable oil, soya beans and walnut) are all good sources of omega-3 fatty acids, which have heart-protective benefits and lower both triglyceride levels and blood pressure. Linolenic, alpha-linolenic, eicosapentaenoic and docosahexaenoic acids are all essential fatty acids.
- **Dietary cholesterol:** Cholesterol is present in food that comes from animals, including poultry, fish, eggs, meats and dairy products.

Although monounsaturated and especially polyunsaturated fats can be helpful in lowering LDL and triglyceride levels, they should still be eaten in moderation. Fats have twice the calories of protein and carbohydrates (9 calories per gram versus approximately 4), and too much of any kind will widen your waistline, no questions.

Less than 10 per cent of daily calories should come from saturated and transunsaturated fats. People with LDL cholesterol of high LDL cholesterol levels may benefit from lowering saturated fat intake even lower (to less than 7 per cent of calories). Two to three servings of oily fish are recommended weekly for the cardioprotective benefits of omega-3 fatty acids.

Fake Fats

Fat substitutes are food additives derived from protein, carbohydrates or chemically modified fat. They are designed to replace the texture, moisture-retention and bulk of fat in food while contributing a lower amount of calories. The main pitfall of reduced-fat and fat-free foods is that some people interpret the label as meaning calorie-free, and overindulge. However, when prudently used, reduced-fat products can be a useful component of a weight-loss plan. Further studies are needed to determine the long-term impact of fat substitutes on overall calorie intake and nutrient absorption.

Food with high fat and/or high protein levels can delay the absorption of carbohydrates, and consequently the postprandial (after meal) rise of blood glucose. People who take insulin need to be especially aware of this phenomenon, as taking insulin too early can result in unwanted highs or lows. Pizza is one food that is well known for causing this 'delayed reaction' in people with diabetes.

Some fat substitutes, such as olestra (Olean), may inhibit the absorption of fat-soluble vitamins A, D, E and K. Olestra has been the subject of much controversy. After 25 years of research, the US Food and Drug Administration (1996) approved olestra as a partial fat replacer. However, the FDA has mandated that products made with olestra be fortified with these vitamins to overcome the deficit. Olestra is not approved for use in the UK (and currently there is no application pending).

Protein and Diabetes

Proteins are chains of amino acids responsible for cell growth and maintenance, and are found in virtually every part of the body. Protein in foods from animal sources (meat, poultry, fish and dairy products) is called complete protein because it contains essential amino acids necessary for building and maintaining cells. Plant-based foods such as grains, beans, fruit and vegetables contain incomplete proteins, with only partial groups of these amino acids. However, different incomplete plant-based proteins can be combined to form complete proteins in the diet. If you are a vegetarian or vegan and have diabetes, a dietician with experience in vegetarian menu planning can advise you on appropriate protein consumption.

Diabetes UK guidelines suggest that people with diabetes should keep their daily protein consumption down to less than 1g per kg body weight. The exception to this is people with impaired kidney function, or nephropathy; these individuals may benefit from a low-protein diet. If you have kidney problems, talk to your doctor and dietician about an appropriate level of protein for your diet.

Sensible Sodium Intake

In moderate amounts, dietary sodium or sodium chloride (salt) is not harmful. In fact, the mineral helps to maintain a healthy electrolyte balance and works in tandem with potassium to regulate blood acid/base balance, heart function, nerve impulses and muscle contractions.

However, people with high blood pressure need to be cautious about having too much sodium in their daily diet. Sodium acts as a vasoconstrictor, constricting (or tightening) blood vessels, which can elevate blood pressure even further. The recommendation for people with diabetes is a sodium chloride intake of not more than 6g per day – that's the equivalent of about one teaspoonful of salt.

When calculating your sodium intake, be sure to include the sodium in processed foods as well as the salt you add to your food. Be on the lookout for monosodium glutamate (MSG), sodium nitrite (nitrate), sodium caseinate, sodium alginate, sodium sulfite, sodium hydroxinate, sodium propionate, sodium saccharin, sodium bicarbonate (bicarbonate of soda) and sodium benzoate. Even some multivitamins contain sodium.

Some people with diabetes and hypertension may benefit from an even bigger cut in dietary salt. A 2001 study published in the American *New England Journal of Medicine* examined sodium intake in the Dietary Approaches to Stop Hypertension (DASH) diet and found that reducing sodium intake to levels below the current recommendation of 2,400 milligrams per day to 1,560 milligrams (65 mmol) and 960 milligrams (40 mmol) reduces blood pressure significantly when it is part of a comprehensive DASH diet – a dietary approach that is low in saturated fat and cholesterol and rich in fibre, protein, calcium, magnesium and potassium.

Chapter 11

Eating Well in Action

If you're looking for a 'diabetic diet' full of bland, boring foods and completely devoid of any desserts, indulgences or the other little taste treats that make life worth living, you are out of luck. The so-called diabetic diet is largely a myth; people with diabetes can and do enjoy a wide variety of foods, the same foods everyone else can eat. The key is moderation, a focus on healthier food choices and a keener awareness of how foods affect your blood glucose levels and your body.

Menu Planning

A meeting with a state registered dietician is an absolute must for anyone with diabetes. You should have access to a hospital-based dietician if there is no community dietician in your area. Sometimes, designated members of the primary care team (at your GP's surgery) are trained in giving dietary advice, but ask your doctor for a referral to a dietician if necessary. A good dietician will explain the mysteries of exchanges and carbohydrate counting to you, and will work with you to create a meal plan that works with your lifestyle. Parents cooking for a child with Type 1 diabetes will have a whole different set of concerns and dietary issues than, for example, an adult with Type 2 who wants to learn how to eat for better control when he's out on the road. If you don't have a dietician already, talk to your doctor about a referral.

As part of your diabetes care team, your dietician should be in close contact with your doctor and diabetes specialist nurse or practice nurse. Make sure she's on top of any adjustments to your insulin or medication, which go hand in hand with what you're eating. The dietician's office is another of those places where it helps to bring a partner or friend for another set of ears, particularly your first time there.

I'm trying hard to manage my Type 2 diabetes through diet and exercise, but my wife continues to buy my favourite junk food for the kids. How can I eat well with that around?
Diabetes is a family disease. Ask your wife to join you for a diabetes education class and/or a meeting with your dietician, and discuss ways of promoting a healthier lifestyle for the entire family. Your children will actually benefit from the same type of healthy meal plan that you're following for your diabetes.

Your dietician will work with you in order to come up with a practical and realistic approach to the dietary management of your diabetes. She will help you to incorporate the healthy eating guidelines into your own meal plans, taking into account your tastes, cultural preferences and so on.

On average you will probably be eating between 45 and 60 per cent of your total daily calories in the form of carbohydrates. A 1,600-calorie diet that is 50 per cent carbohydrates, for example, would be 800 calories from carbohydrates. Since 1g of carbohydrate has an energy value of 4 calories, this equates to a daily carbohydrate intake of about 200g. Your dietician will probably advise you to spread out your carbohydrate intake throughout the day to promote better blood glucose control.

Low-carb, high-protein diets have soared in popularity thanks to medical media icons like the late Dr Atkins. However, the jury is still out on their long-term safety. People with kidney impairment should avoid any diet that is heavy on protein, as it can worsen the condition. If you'd like to try a lower-carb meal plan, talk with your dietician and your doctor about a safe approach that's right for you.

A Healthy Plateful

Diabetes UK recommends that people with diabetes should eat a healthy, balanced diet, just like the rest of the population.

What's a healthy, balanced diet? Food is divided into five main types or groups, and the 'plate model' is used to help illustrate how much of the foods from each of the groups we should be eating. Imagine a plate divided into three: one third full of fruit and vegetables, another third full of starchy foods, and the other third for the dairy, meat and fat/sugar groups.

No food is 'bad' or 'forbidden' – just keep the portions sensible.

Fruit and vegetables
Apples, oranges, pears, bananas, mangoes, fruit juice, lettuce, tomatoes, spinach, broccoli
Starchy foods
Bread, cereals, oats, potatoes, pasta, noodles, rice

Dairy products
Milk, cheese, yoghurt
Meat and high-protein foods
Lean meat, poultry, fish, pulses, nuts
Foods containing fat and/or sugar
Butter, margarine, oils, salad dressings, crisps, cakes, biscuits, pastries,
puddings, chocolate, sweets

Dear Diary...

Even if you follow your meal plan to the letter, you're still going to find
that certain foods will give you a bigger spike in glucose levels than
expected. You may also find that other foods you expected to bump up
your readings barely affect them. That's the individual nature of
diabetes. For this reason, a food diary is an invaluable tool in working
out just how different foods affect your blood glucose levels.

Record the type, amount and timing of foods eaten, along with
what affect they had on your blood glucose levels (a reading before
eating and a reading two hours after eating). Many people choose to
record the information in their blood glucose logbook. At first it
may feel a little obsessive-compulsive to chronicle every bite, but
you'll find it's worth it when the time comes to work out a
mysterious high or an unexpected low. It's also a great cure for
mindless eating – you won't be polishing off what the kids left on
their dinner plate or munching samples in the supermarket if you've
trained yourself to write it down.

Carbohydrate Counting

Carbohydrate counting, in its various forms, has been around the block
a few times. Its importance is mostly for people using insulin to control
their blood glucose levels. Carbohydrate counting involves calculating
the grams of carbohydrate eaten in a given meal or snack.

In the past, a strict carbohydrate diet would be prescribed – 40g for
breakfast, 50g for lunch and 60g for dinner, with 10 or 20g snacks

between meals, for example. Set insulin doses then 'covered' the carbohydrate intake. This very structured approach was then phased out in the UK, in favour of more general, less specific, healthy eating guidelines. However, carbohydrate counting is now coming back into vogue, with a much more flexible approach to diet and insulin dosing.

How many carbohydrates you eat in a given day depends on your unique caloric, medical and lifestyle needs. An active teenager will have a greater carbohydrate requirement than an inactive adult. Again, the first step in establishing a carbohydrate-counting plan is sitting down with a registered dietician who will discuss your medical history, lifestyle, eating habits and medication routines, and come up with a plan for how many carbohydrates you should be eating and when they should be consumed.

As you learn how variations in food choices, timing of meals and exercise affect your blood glucose levels, you and your dietician and doctor can work together to fine-tune your carbohydrate-counting approch for optimal control.

How Much in What

You can use a reference book to find out the carbohydrate values of most foods. Utilize the labelling information on packaged foods – carbohydrate values are typically given per 100g as well as per serving (be careful to see exactly what counts as a serving!).

My dietician told me that 15g of carbohydrate is equal to one serving, but that doesn't always match the serving size information on the food labels I read. Which is right?
Both! For example, a half-cup of apple juice has 15g of carbohydrates and is equivalent to one carb choice serving, but the carbohydrates for the serving size indicated on the label would be twice that (30g, or two carbohydrate choice servings). Make sure you know how many carbs you are consuming in your serving size.

Advanced Carbohydrate Counting

Carbohydrate counting can offer people who use insulin more control and greater flexibility in what they eat. If you use a fast-acting insulin such as Humalog or NovoRapid prior to a meal, you can determine how many units you need to take, based on both your blood glucose reading prior to the meal and on the number of carbohydrate grams you plan on eating. This is referred to as 'covering' your carbohydrates.

Usually, the starting point for this insulin-to-carbohydrate ratio is about 1 unit of insulin for every 10–15g of carbohydrates on the menu. People who are more insulin-resistant tend to require a larger amount of insulin to cover a certain amount of carbohydrate, compared to those who are more insulin-sensitive. By monitoring your blood glucose levels and noting responses to different amounts and types of carbohydrates, you and your diabetes specialist should be able to fine-tune your own specific insulin-to-carbohydrate ratios.

Insulin pump users learn the ins and outs of advanced carbohydrate counting as part of their training in pump therapy. This approach to diet also forms the basis of DAFNE – dose adjustment for normal eating – a five-day structured education programme that teaches people with Type 1 diabetes how to adjust insulin to accommodate their lifestyle and food choices from day to day.

People who are more insulin-resistant may require a larger amount of insulin than those who still retain a great deal of insulin sensitivity. There are several methods for computing insulin sensitivity and insulin-to-carbohydrate ratio; for more information, see Chapter 8.

Glycaemic Index (GI)

While carbohydrate counting is based on the idea that all carbohydrates are created equal, and it is the total number of carbohydrate grams, not the type of carohydrate (i.e. simple or complex; starch or fruit) that is the bottom line for blood glucose control, the glycaemic index takes a different tack, looking at carbohydrate quality instead of quantity.

The GI is a measure of how quickly a carbohydrate affects blood glucose levels. High-GI foods cause quick spikes, while low-GI foods provide a slower, steadier release of glucose. In general, unprocessed, fibre-rich foods tend to be the lowest on the GI scale, while processed and starch-heavy carbohydrates are the highest.

To determine the glycaemic index of a food, researchers give a test subject some quantity of the food that contains 50g of carbohydrates, and their blood glucose levels are then measured at regular intervals to determine how quickly the carbohydrates in the food turn into glucose. That response is then measured against a standard value of how quickly 50g of either glucose or white bread (both 100 on the GI scale) causes blood glucose to rise, and is expressed as a percentage between 1 and 140. The results among a group of testers (usually ten) are averaged to come up with the GI.

Using the GI

Some people with diabetes use the GI as a reference guide for choosing slow, low-GI carbohydrates to keep glucose levels under control and avoid blood sugar spikes. High-GI foods also have their place. If you're about to go for a quick sprint, you'd want to make sure a pre-exercise carbohydrate snack provides the quick release of energy you need. And a fast-acting, high GI carbohydrate is preferable over a low one for treating a hypo.

One important caveat to using the GI as your guide – don't become so carbohydrate-centric that you lose sight of your overall nutrient intake. The lower-GI food may not always be the best choice; a Snickers bar has a GI of 44, while a bowl of Cheerios has a GI of 74. Although this may be your perfect justification for satisfying your sweet tooth, it's obvious that the healthier choice here is the cereal. Keep your vitamins, minerals, protein and fat intake in perspective.

Glycaemic Load

Another anomaly of the GI is that the system doesn't make adjustments for the quantity of carbohydrates per serving. Some foods with a high index value simply don't contain enough carbohydrates per serving to make much of an impact on glucose levels. You'd have to eat over six servings of cooked beets to get the same amount of carbohydrates in one large baked potato, yet both have a relatively high GI (91 and 121, respectively).

Researchers at the Harvard School of Public Health in the USA have come up with a way to bridge this quality versus quantity gap – the *glycaemic load*. To work out the glycaemic load of a food, convert its GI percentage value into decimal format (i.e. 91 is equivalent to .91) and multiply it by the grams of carbohydrates in one serving. At first glance, you might want to pass up beetroot based on their GI alone, despite the fact that it is an excellent source of folate and potassium. But although the GI of cooked beetroot is 91, a 30g serving only has 8.46g of carbohydrates. That makes its glycaemic load only 7.69 (.91 x 8.46). By comparison, a carbohydrate-dense large baked potato has 50.96 carbohydrates (with skin), a GI of 121 and a whopping glycaemic load of 62.

Food GI is not set in stone. Raw foods may have a different GI than the same food cooked; preparation methods can also affect GI. Fruits may have a lower or higher GI depending on their stage of ripeness. Some foods will not have a GI, and it isn't unusual for the GI of processed foods to vary by brand. In addition, one version of GI uses white bread for the reference food, while the other uses glucose.

It's Not Easy

GI is a good tool for making smart food choices. However, it does require a motivated patient who isn't scared of a little maths. And because GI is not something listed on food labels, it requires a small investment in a book of GI listings. Drs Jennie Brand-Miller and Thomas Wolever are considered two of the world's leading authorities on the GI, and have written what is arguably the best book of the bunch – *The New Glucose Revolution*. There are also several lists and GI databases available online (see Appendix A for more information).

In the recently published nutritional guidelines from Diabetes UK, the utility of the Glycaemic Index was noted, with the recommendation that carbohydrate foods with a low GI should be more actively promoted. If you want to know more about using the GI, talk with your dietician about how best to incorporate it into your meal plan.

Weights and Measures

You can't measure every morsel that passes your lips, but it can be helpful to measure most foods and beverages until you get a feel for portion sizes. It's a supersized world out there, and most people are surprised to find that their idea of a single serving is actually two or three.

A Rough Idea

Get intimate with your food, or rather, your dishes. Do you have a favourite mug or bowl? Pay attention to how completely a serving of yoghurt or soup fills it up. You'll soon that find it's second nature to guesstimate your portion sizes.

There will be times when you can't use your favourite cup; bringing it to a restaurant is a little unrealistic. In these cases, it helps to have some rough equivalents for comparison.

Here are some typical serving sizes and some points of reference for estimating portion sizes:

- 250ml of yoghurt – a clenched fist or a small apple
- 90g (3oz) of fish, meat or poultry – a pack of cards, the palm of your hand or a pocket pack of tissues
- One teaspoon of butter or mayonnaise – a thimble, a thumb tip (top knuckle to tip) or the head of a toothbrush
- 30g (1oz) of cheese – your entire thumb, a tube of lip salve or an AA battery

Using your hands to estimate servings is probably the easiest method – you don't leave home without them. However, make sure you compare your hand amounts against food that has been measured out until you get a sense of how accurately you're estimating. Of course, if you have particularly large or small hands, you need to adjust for size.

Even for the more experienced portion predictor, it's a good idea to test your skills at least once a month and measure your guess at a serving size. It's easy to start overdoing it, and the little bits (and bites) add up. If your control has been off for no apparent reason, one of the first things to check is whether your serving sizes are on target.

Eating Out

Some restaurants are notorious for serving up helpings well beyond a single serving size. To keep your intake under control, you can split a main course, order from the starter menu, or simply eat half and take half home. In some restaurants, you may be able to order a child-size portion (but even some children's menu items may be larger than a single serving). Ask your server to serve condiments on the side so your food isn't swimming in sauce, and stay away from the bread basket, chips or complimentary snacks if you're fond of munching mindlessly.

Many national restaurant chains, particularly fast-food establishments, will provide nutritional and serving size information on menu items upon request. Ask your waiter, or look online.

When planning a meal out, don't set yourself up for failure. Choose a place that you know offers some food choices that will fit in to your meal plan. If you must meet at the local greasy spoon, where lard is a food group, fill up on a healthy meal at home first. If you're on the road or in unfamiliar territory, don't be afraid to phone first or ask to see a menu at the door before committing yourself to a restaurant choice. Ask questions about ingredients and preparation methods. If you feel a need to explain why you won't be eating somewhere, tell the hostess you're on a special diet. Some establishments may offer to prepare a dish in an alternate way (e.g. steaming instead of frying it) that isn't on the standard menu to keep your patronage.

When Temptation Strikes

You've had a delicious yet healthy meal and are feeling pleased with yourself for turning down the bacon double cheeseburger that had been calling your name for broiled fish and steamed vegetables. And then the torture device rolls into view – a sweets trolley laden with trays of your favourite cheesecake, fudge cake, and apple tart with cream. You can feel your blood glucose rising just looking at it.

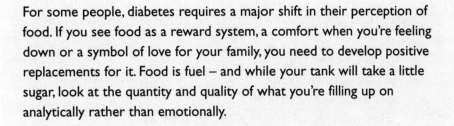

For some people, diabetes requires a major shift in their perception of food. If you see food as a reward system, a comfort when you're feeling down or a symbol of love for your family, you need to develop positive replacements for it. Food is fuel – and while your tank will take a little sugar, look at the quantity and quality of what you're filling up on analytically rather than emotionally.

You can say 'to hell with it!' and order the richest slab of carbohydrates on the trolley; grin and bear it while your dining companion savours his slice of banoffie pie and ice-cream; or use the situation as an opportunity to practise moderation. You will not be struck by lightning if you indulge occasionally, provided your splurges are built into your overall meal plan. Split a small dessert with a friend, or ask for half now and half in a doggy bag. If the offerings are truly too rich for your blood, promise yourself a frozen yoghurt or another treat on your way home. Don't deny yourself – it's not an all-or-nothing game. In fact, the stress of doing so constantly may raise your blood glucose levels higher than the occasional chocolate fudge brownie.

Social occasions that are centred around eating, such as a birthday party, a holiday gathering or a family reunion barbeque, offer a whole new set of challenges. Well-meaning friends and relatives frequently feel the need to be the food police, asking with every pass of the plate, 'Should you be eating that?' The best answer is simple: 'Most people with diabetes can eat just about anything you can, in moderation. I have a few books you can borrow that explain more if you're interested.' Ideally, they'll take you up on your offer and learn a thing or two. If they don't, you've probably stopped them from pestering you, at least until Christmas. Chapter 21 has more suggestions for handling food and special occasions.

Smart Snack Substitutes

Even though you can indulge occasionally, if you've made a regular habit of junk food, it's one you'll have to kick. Still, having many small meals or minisnacks between meals can be beneficial to keeping blood glucose on an even keel, and your dietician will work these into your meal plan.

Cut out the fatty fried snacks, sugary drinks and sugar-encrusted snack pies, and try some of these healthier snack choices instead:

- fresh or dried fruit
- crackers, crispbreads
- unsweetened cereal
- wholemeal or wholegrain bread, rolls, toast
- use raw vegetables and salad
- use nuts and/or seeds (sparingly!) for variety
- choose low fat spreads.

Regaining Control After a Fall

If you haven't already, at one point in your life you will probably end up with an 'Oh, no!' reading after splurging on something you shouldn't have. Ask yourself if there was a specific trigger for the slip-up, such as a particularly stressful day at work or going to a party hungry. If you can pinpoint a cause, think about how you can prevent it from happening next time, whether it be by adjusting your eating schedule or by learning some stress-management techniques.

It is not the end of the world if you mess up. If you're too busy kicking yourself, you'll miss any lesson you might gain from your mistake. Diabetes is a disease of highs and lows, both physically and emotionally. Strive to achieve balance in the emotional area – as well as the physical one.

Chapter 12

Don't Forget to Exercise!

One of the simplest and most effective ways to bring down blood glucose levels, cut the risk of cardiovascular disease and improve overall health and well-being is exercise. Yet in our increasingly sedentary world, where almost every essential task can be performed online, from the driver's seat or with a phone call, exercising can be a hard approach to sell.

The Importance of Exercise

The research evidence is clear. People who are physically active reduce their risk of developing major chronic diseases (such as heart disease and diabetes) by a whopping 50 per cent. Just 30 minutes of physical activity each day is recommended for the adult population in order to maintain good general health. Inactivity is thought to be one of the key reasons for the surge of Type 2 diabetes, because inactivity and obesity promote insulin resistance.

The good news is that it's never too late to get moving, and exercise is one of the easiest ways to start controlling your diabetes. For people with Type 2 diabetes in particular, exercise can improve insulin sensitivity, lower the risk of heart disease, and promote weight loss.

A 2003 animal study published in the *Journal of Clinical Endocrinology and Metabolism* found that lack of exercise – and not diet – was the key factor behind obesity and diabetes. The findings suggest that exercise may play an even bigger role than previously thought in diabetes control and prevention in humans.

While several studies have demonstrated that regular exercise can lower HbA1c (average long-term glucose) levels in Type 2 diabetes, more research is needed to firmly establish that link. At the time of writing, there was no clinical data supporting a long-term HbA1c-lowering effect in Type 1 diabetes. But despite the lack of conclusive scientific evidence, exercise still has many benefits for people with Type 1 diabetes, including improved blood cholesterol levels, lower blood pressure, better heart health and the short-term suppression of blood glucose levels.

Getting Started

The first order of business with any exercise plan, especially if you're a dyed-in-the-wool couch potato, is to consult your health care provider. If you have cardiac risk factors, she may want to perform a stress test to establish a safe level of exercise for you.

Certain diabetic complications will also dictate what type of exercise programme you can take on. Activities such as weightlifting, jogging or high-impact aerobics can possibly pose a risk for people with diabetic retinopathy due to the risk of further blood vessel damage and possible retinal detachment. Patients with severe peripheral neuropathy (PN) should avoid foot-intensive weight-bearing exercises, such as long-distance walking, jogging or step aerobics, and opt instead for low-impact activities such as swimming, cycling and rowing. If you have conditions that make exercise a challenge, your doctor may refer you to an exercise physiologist or physiotherapist, who can design a fitness programme for your specific needs.

If you're already active in sports or work out regularly, it will still benefit you to discuss your regular routine with your doctor. If you're taking insulin, you may need to take special precautions to prevent hypoglycaemia during your workout.

Start Slowly

Your exercise routine can be as simple as a brisk nightly neighbourhood walk. If you haven't been very active before now, start slowly and work your way up. Walk the dog or get out in the garden and rake the leaves. Take the stairs instead of the lift or escalator. Park in the back of the car park and walk. Every little bit does, in fact, help.

Leg pain during exercise, especially aching in the calves, buttocks or thighs, could be intermittent claudication and peripheral vascular disease (a potential complication of diabetes). Doctor-supervised exercise, particularly walking, can actually help ease the pain over time. Medication may also be required.

As little as 15–30 minutes of daily, heart-pumping exercise can make a big difference in your blood glucose control and your risk of developing diabetic complications. One of the easiest and least expensive ways of getting moving is to start a walking programme. All you need is a good pair of well-fitting, supportive shoes and a direction to walk.

Do pay particular attention to your feet both before and after you walk or run. Because of the risk of foot ulcers and other diabetic foot problems, you should examine them carefully for blisters and abrasions and treat them promptly if they do occur. Seamless, waterproof socks that take moisture away from your feet can help to prevent friction while walking. For more on diabetic foot care, see Chapter 16.

Making Time

Everyone is busy. But considering what's at stake, making time for exercise needs to be a priority right now. Thirty minutes a day isn't much, when you come down to it. Cut one sitcom out of your evening television viewing schedule. Get up half an hour earlier each morning. Use half of your lunch hour for a brisk walk. You can find the time if you look hard enough for it.

You don't have to spend a lot of money on expensive health club memberships, treadmills or the latest fitness gadgets to get moving. However, some people find that if they make a monetary investment, they're more likely to follow through on fitness. If you don't have a lot of money to spend, find out about a basic membership at a local gym, fitness club or community centre.

You can also try combining exercise with something else already on your schedule. If you normally spend an hour on Saturday morning playing video games with your kids, get away from virtual reality and play a real game of football or Frisbee outside. Get off the riding mower and cut the grass the old-fashioned way – with a manual push mower. Wake up early and walk your kids to school. Look for opportunities rather than excuses.

Exercise Intensity

How hard you should be pushing yourself depends on your level of fitness and your health history. Your doctor can recommend an optimal heart rate target for working out based on these factors. On average, most people should aim for a target heart rate zone of 50–75 per cent of your maximum heart rate. Maximum heart rate is computed by subtracting your age from the number 220. So if you are 40, your maximum heart rate would be 180, and your target heart rate zone would be between 90 and 135 beats per minute.

You should wear a digital or analog watch with a second hand or function to check your heart rate during exercise. You can calculate heart rate by placing your fingers at your wrist or neck pulse point and counting the number of beats for 15 seconds. Multiply that number by four to get your heart rate.

The number you get should be within your target zone. If it's too high, take your intensity down a few notches. If you're exercising below your target zone, pick things up. If you are new to exercise, you should aim for the lower (50 per cent) range of your target heart rate. As you become more fit, you can work towards the 75 per cent maximum.

Exercise and Blood Glucose Levels

When you exercise, your body uses glucose for energy. During the first 15 minutes of your workout routine, your body converts the glycogen stored in your muscles back into glucose, and also uses the glucose circulating in your bloodstream for fuel. This action causes the natural blood-glucose-lowering effect of exercise.

After 15 minutes, your body turns to the liver to convert its glycogen stockpile into glucose energy. After about 30 minutes, your cells will also begin to burn free fatty acids (FFA) for fuel. Once the glycogen stores are used up, without a carbohydrate refuelling in the form of food, hypoglycaemia is a real danger, particularly in those with Type 1 diabetes.

Before you get moving, test your glucose levels. If they are less than 6.0 mmol/l, don't start working out without a carbohydrate snack for fuel. Some fast-acting carbohydrate (such as Lucozade) should be available during and after your workout, in case you need it.

Exercise and Snacking

Because of the risk of hypoglycaemia during exercise, especially in Type 1 diabetes, a pre-exercise snack may be required. How much of a snack and when to eat it depends on your blood glucose readings and the planned intensity and duration of your workout. In general, people with Type 2 diabetes who work out at a moderate level will probably not require a snack before exercise, particularly if they are trying to lose weight.

For people with Type 1 diabetes, moderately intense exercise lasting longer than 30 minutes will probably require a snack of at least 15g of carbohydrates. If you're planning on a high-energy game of squash that may last an hour or more, you will need a bigger carb boost of between 25 and 50g of carbohydrates. Adding protein and/or fat to the carbohydrates can extend the glucose action over time if you're embarking on a long-distance bike ride or similar activity. A snack should be taken about 15–30 minutes before exercise for the best results.

If you're going on a low-intensity, half-hour walk and your glucose readings are at least 6.0 mmol/l, you may not need any extra carbohydrates (although you should bring some with you just in case).

Keeping an exercise log along with your blood glucose readings can help you determine what works best for you. Different sports and routines will have diverse effects on your blood glucose levels. Discuss your exercise plans with your diabetes care team to find out the best routine for preparing for exercise.

Never exercise immediately following a regular meal, and don't plan exercise during the time your insulin is peaking. Exercise can cause injected insulin to work much faster because your circulation is speeded up as your heart pumps harder. In many cases, you may need to adjust your insulin dose downwards for those times you will be exercising; again, your doctor or diabetes specialist nurse can offer you further advice on what's right for your situation.

Lows (Hypoglycaemia)

If you start to feel a hypo coming on, don't panic. Stop exercising and test immediately. If your levels are too low, eat or drink 15g of fast-acting carbohydrate right away. Don't resume your workout. Wait 15 minutes for the carbohydrates to kick in and test again. If your levels are still too low, take 15 more grams and follow the same routine until blood glucose levels are back in a normal range.

A glucose gel or glucose tablet is a good choice for a fast-acting carbohydrate. Both are compact enough to carry along while you exercise and work quickly. Invest in a waterproof bum bag to keep both your glucose gel/tablets and testing supplies in during your workout.

After your workout is finished, your body will recharge its energy stores by processing your blood glucose into glycogen. Depending on the level of exercise intensity and the amount of glycogen that needs to be replaced, this process could take anywhere from four to 24 hours. This is why post-exercise glucose testing is important, as hypoglycaemia can occur well after you've finished exercising.

Highs (Hyperglycaemia)

In some cases, when blood glucose levels are high and insulin levels are low to begin with, the adrenaline rush from heavy exercise can have the opposite effect, signalling the liver and muscles to break down glycogen into glucose. In these cases, ketoacidosis is a danger.

If your blood sugars test high before exercise, *always* test for ketones before you start your workout. If your levels are high and you do choose to exercise, make sure you test glucose levels again about 15 minutes into your workout to ensure they are coming back down.

Take Precautions

To avoid dangerous highs and lows during exercise, make sure you take the precautions outlined overleaf.

- **Test first.** Always take a blood glucose reading before your workout.
- **Warm up.** Always stretch out before exercising to avoid injury, and start your routine with five to ten minutes of low-intensity movement.
- **Wet down.** Drink plenty of fluids before, during, and after your workout to prevent dehydration. If you're exercising in the heat, drink even more.
- **Cool off.** If you're working out intensely, take it down a few notches at a time, and spend five to ten minutes bringing your heart rate back down to its pre-workout level.
- **Carb load.** Have a fast-acting carbohydrate on hand in case of hypoglycaemia, and don't hesitate to use it.
- **Test last.** Once your workout is over, test your blood glucose levels again to ensure they aren't dipping too low.

You should always wear or carry medical identification, but it's particularly important when you are exercising. Before you go for that run, make sure you are wearing your ID in a visible location. A shoelace tag or watchband ID are sports-friendly options if you find that your usual ID bracelet or necklace gets in the way of your workout.

Everyone Can Exercise

Virtually everyone who has the capability to move can exercise to some degree. Even if you suffer from complications related to your diabetes or other health conditions, your doctor can recommend a level and form of exercise that is appropriate for you.

Chances are that you already work out without even knowing it. Things you have never considered 'exercise', like washing the car or cleaning your house, are actually calorie-burning, heart-pumping ways to get fit. All the following activities will burn about 150 calories a day (or 1,000 calories a week):

- Washing and waxing a car for 45 to 60 minutes
- Washing windows or floors for 45 to 60 minutes

- Gardening for 30–45 minutes
- Pushing a buggy 2.5km (1.5 miles) in 30 minutes
- Raking leaves for 30 minutes
- Walking 3km (2 miles) in 30 minutes (15 minutes per 1.5km/1 mile)
- Doing water aerobics for 30 minutes
- Bicycling 6km (4 miles) in 15 minutes
- Shovelling snow for 15 minutes
- Climbing steps for 15 minutes.

Disabled and Chronically Ill

For people with orthopaedic conditions, joint pain or musculoskeletal problems, low-impact exercise is usually the best bet. Swimming is a good low-impact form of resistance exercise. If you are in a wheelchair or unable to stand or stay on your feet for long periods of time without support, chair exercises may also be a good option.

Dealing with Obesity

If you are extremely overweight or obese, exercise is especially important, yet it can present unique challenges. Comfort is an issue; certain exercises, such as jogging and high-impact aerobics, may simply not be feasible. Weight lies heavy on the mind as well as the body, and it's possible you may not be feeling mentally or emotionally prepared to join group or team exercises.

Work on your own level. Don't try step aerobics just yet. Contact your local gym, fitness club or community centre to see if there's a 'plus-size' exercise programme available. And always check with your doctor before starting a new fitness routine. A referral to a physiotherapist may be appropriate, particularly if you have other health problems.

It may be easier said than done, but don't feel self-conscious. If you feel uncomfortable amid all the Lycra and rippling abs at the local health club, then don't torture yourself – find an environment that you feel at ease in. Try a walking programme, either outside or at home on a treadmill. The impact-free environment of a swimming pool is also a good place to start getting fit. Team up with a friend and motivate each other. Exercise should make you feel good about yourself. Every step you take is a step towards a healthier you.

Exercising for the Elderly

Staying active is particularly important as you grow older. Ageing is associated with increased insulin resistance, and it's thought that this is at least partially attributable to a loss of muscle mass. Keep on track with an active lifestyle and strength-training exercises to retain muscle mass and insulin sensitivity. It's never too late to get moving. Talk to your doctor today about an appropriate exercise programme that promotes strength, balance, flexibility and endurance.

Get Your Kids to Exercise, Too

Children with Type 1 diabetes are probably the least likely to need motivation to exercise. After all, most parents have a harder time keeping kids quiet than getting them moving. Yet because of often unpredictable blood glucose levels, particularly in younger children, they also are the group that probably requires the most vigilance in monitoring to avoid exercise-induced hypoglycaemia. They also play hard, so testing should be frequent even in the absence of structured sports or exercise.

My daughter has Type 1 diabetes and wants to join a local football team. Should I let her?

By all means! Children with diabetes should be encouraged to take part in the same activities as their peers. However, coaches and other adults who oversee your child's participation in team or individual sports should be educated about the signs and treatment of hypoglycaemia.

For overweight children or adolescents with Type 2 diabetes, or those who are considered at risk for the disease, exercise is absolutely imperative for all the reasons previously cited for adults – weight loss, improved insulin sensitivity and overall health and well-being.

Staying Motivated

One of the biggest obstacles to staying on track for fitness is losing motivation. People who are just starting an exercise programme can find themselves quickly tiring of the same routine. Keeping exercise appealing and maintaining a good fitness perspective is key to long-term success.

Boredom Busters

If you had to watch exactly the same episode of your favourite television show every day for the rest of your life, you'd probably be banging your head against the wall by the end of the week. You'd change the channel, pick up a book or do anything you could to avoid something you once enjoyed. Yet many people starting on a fitness programme feel compelled to follow the same routine day after day after day, and consequently fall off the exercise wagon due to sheer boredom. Try these strategies for keeping your workouts interesting.

- **Mix and match.** Play squash with a friend one week and try water polo the next.
- **Team up.** Get a walking partner or an exercise friend to keep you motivated (and vice versa).
- **Join a team.** Find a local exercise or aerobics group. Even when you aren't feeling much like exercising, your commitment to other team members may get you moving.
- **Relocate.** If you like to cycle, walk or jog, try a new route or area.
- **Go for the goal.** Set new fitness targets for yourself.
- **Reward yourself.** When you reach a new goal, pat yourself on the back with a non-edible reward.
- **Make some noise.** Forget the radio and your CDs, and customize your own soundtrack for working out.
- **Be well read.** Exercise your mind as well as your body with an audiobook.
- **Sound off.** Try it without the Walkman for once, and enjoy the sounds of nature and the neighbourhood.

If you or someone you know is at risk for developing Type 2 diabetes, getting fit can help. The Diabetes Prevention Trial found that minor lifestyle changes, including just 30 minutes of exercise daily, cut the risk of developing Type 2 diabetes in high-risk subjects by 58 per cent.

Keeping it in Perspective

Many people, particularly those with Type 2 diabetes, start exercising for the sole purpose of losing weight. When the pounds don't drop as quickly or as completely as they'd like, they get discouraged and give up. If you take away any message about exercise and diabetes, let it be this: even if you don't lose weight, your investment in exercise is still paying off in reduced heart disease risk and better blood glucose control. And exercise simply makes you feel better, both physically and mentally. Your energy level will rise, and the endorphins released by your brain during exercise will boost your sense of well-being and may help fight diabetes-related depression. Don't give up before you really get started. You owe it to yourself to keep going.

The GP Referral Scheme

The GP Referral Scheme is a relatively new initiative in which GPs give patients an 'exercise prescription'. The idea is that those people who would gain some health benefit from increasing their level of physical activity are given easy access to local facilities such as a swimming pool or gym. In addition, patients are given a basic fitness assessment, and a personal exercise programme is drawn up for you. Close monitoring and lots of encouragement will help you to keep going.

The schemes vary across the country, but the principles are the same, and they are usually the result of a collaboration between the primary health care providers and the local council.

Professional Sports

What do legendary Olympic Gold Medallist Sir Steve Redgrave and famous footballer of the 1980s Gary Mabbutt have in common? They have managed to balance diabetes with a successful professional sports career. That's no small accomplishment given everything you've just learned about insulin, exercise and blood glucose control.

With the exception of a pie-eating contest, there is virtually no competitive event that well-controlled Type 1 or Type 2 diabetes can exclude you from. But professional sportspeople with diabetes must have exemplary self-management skills and be very attuned to their reactions to different levels of activity. They must be as dedicated to blood glucose control as they are to their sport of choice.

Team sports in particular require a coaching staff and team members who are flexible about treatment breaks for blood glucose checks and other essentials. For the most successful relationship, team members and leaders should also be educated about the needs of people with diabetes and the signs and treatment of a hypo.

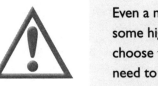

Even a mild episode of hypoglycaemia could have lethal consequences in some high-risk sports such as scuba-diving or rock-climbing. Athletes who choose to participate in sports that demand a high level of concentration need to have a partner familiar with the symptoms of a blood glucose low to ensure safety.

Whether your goal is professional athletics or just a friendly game in the park, working closely with your health care team and remaining aware of the signals your body sends is the best way to attain it.

Chapter 13

Tackling Weight Loss

At least 80 per cent of people with Type 2 diabetes are overweight. In fact, the UK as a nation has been packing on the pounds for the past two decades. One fifth of men and one quarter of women in England are now classified as being obese. In the five years between 1996 and 2001, the number of obese children (6–15 years) rose by 3.5 per cent. Losing weight is one of the best ways to treat Type 2 diabetes, but it is also possibly the most difficult. In addition, people with Type 1 diabetes have to deal with special insulin-related weight problems of their own.

In Control but Gaining Weight

People with Type 1 diabetes face a unique challenge with weight. Frequently, when they start getting their blood glucose levels under control with insulin injections, their weight goes up. When blood glucose levels are high, your body becomes dehydrated, and as your blood glucose levels come under control and your fluid balance returns, you gain water weight.

This is actually a positive development when it occurs shortly after diagnosis; this weight gain helps you recover weight you may have lost leading up to diagnosis.

Better control sometimes comes at the cost of some extra weight. The Diabetes Control and Complications Trial (DCCT) found that as blood glucose levels in Type 1 diabetes came down to normal levels, subjects gained an average of 4.5kg (10lb).

The Role of Insulin

Injected insulin is also helping your body to utilize glucose energy from food. Before you started treatment for your Type 1 diabetes, you may have found that you could eat virtually anything to try to quiet your ravenous hyperglycaemia-induced appetite, and you would not gain any weight. Now that you actually have the insulin to help process the glucose, you'll gain weight, a sign that you're also gaining control over your diabetes. It may also take a while for you to get your appetite back in sync with your newfound control, which can also cause extra weight gain.

Don't get too discouraged by weight gain that occurs with the start of insulin treatment. Again, it's usually a sign that you're getting better, not bigger. If you continue to gain weight or become concerned about the weight you've gained so far, a strategy session with your doctor and dietician is in order. They may be able to recommend dietary and insulin adjustments that can help bring unwanted weight gain to a halt. Sometimes a switch to a different insulin type or an insulin pump can help you to get a handle on weight fluctuations.

Type 2 and Insulin

People with Type 2 diabetes who switch to insulin injections to achieve better control over their blood sugars can also find themselves gaining weight. If you are Type 2 and are already overweight or obese, weight gain can increase your insulin resistance, which in turn will increase your insulin dose requirement. It's essential to talk to your doctor about possible adjustments to treatment before you find yourself in a vicious cycle of insulin resistance and weight gain.

Type 2 Medications and Weight Gain

Some of the hypoglycaemic drugs prescribed for Type 2 diabetes can cause weight gain as well. Insulin-sensitizing thiazolidinediones (also called TZDs or glitizones), including Actos (pioglitazone) and Avandia (rosiglitazone), and sulphonylurea drugs, fall into this category. Because glitizones can also cause oedema, weight gain from their use may mean a gain in fluids rather than fat. On the flip side, metformin can cause weight loss in some people.

Weight Loss and Type 2 Diabetes

The Diabetes Prevention Program (DPP), carried out in the USA, proved that even modest weight loss can prevent or delay the onset of Type 2 diabetes in overweight at-risk adults. But what about people who already have the disease? The news is good for you as well. Weight loss can reduce your need for medication and insulin, improve your cardiovascular health and, best of all, it will make you feel good about yourself.

Weight and Insulin Resistance

Precisely how excess fat promotes insulin resistance isn't yet entirely clear, but it is thought that certain proteins and/or enzymes released by stored fat act on muscle and liver cells to impair the way that they 'read' insulin signals to process glucose.

In addition, research has found that the 'apple-shaped' body (central abdominal obesity) associated with insulin resistance and Type 2 diabetes contains fat with unique properties. Specifically, this type of visceral abdominal fat sheds more free fatty acids, which can elevate triglyceride levels, and is associated with higher insulin levels that promote further fat storage. Paring down your abdominal fat has the double benefit of both increasing insulin sensitivity and decreasing triglyceride levels in people with Type 2 diabetes.

According to the government and data from the Health Survey for England, in 2002, 22 per cent of adults were obese (BMI >30). Women were slightly more likely to be obese than men (25 per cent compared with 23 per cent). However, more men than women were in the overweight category (BMI 25–30; 43 per cent compared with 33 per cent). Combining the overweight and obese groups, approximately two-thirds of men and half of women are either overweight or obese. There is also a higher prevalence of obesity among certain ethnic groups, and particularly among Black Caribbean and Pakistani women.

Shedding Wisely

First and foremost, you need a plan that dovetails with your diabetes management programme. Book a date with your dietician so you can strategize on meal plans to promote weight loss. Talk to your doctor before embarking on any new exercise plan so she can assess your heart health and give your workout her official stamp of approval.

If you have diabetic complications or other health issues that affect your mobility, an exercise physiologist and/or physiotherapist may be able to help get you on track with a low-impact or adaptive exercise programme.

Set Realistic Goals

Many people end up abandoning perfectly good weight-loss programmes before they even lace up their trainers. Why? Because in a world filled with fast food, instant messaging and five-second glucose meters, anything without a quick payoff goes against the grain of the prevalent Western instant gratification ethic. While it would be nice to 'lose inches in days!' as the miracle advertisements proclaim, weight loss is a slow and (hopefully) steady process that takes time and commitment.

Setting weight-loss goals for yourself can be a good motivator. Gradual weight loss is usually the safest. A diet that cuts your normal calorie consumption (for your weight) by 500 per day will encourage weight loss. So will burning 500 or more calories each day with exercise. Your best bet is to strike a balance between the two, and make exercise – be it team sports, cycling or walking – something you enjoy and want to continue with. Making a long-term healthy lifestyle change is essential to keeping the weight off once it's gone.

Aim Low

If you wear a size 14 and you spend a bundle on a designer size 8 dress as motivation, you'll probably end up feeling guilty, frustrated and angry if you aren't slinking around in it a month later. You'll do much better setting smaller, achievable targets for yourself. If you must try the new-clothes strategy, go down a size at a time, and don't buy anything you have to take out a second mortgage to pay for.

The latest government data (2002) suggest that in England, over one in five boys and over one in four girls aged 2–15 are either overweight or obese. Childhood obesity is leading to to an alarming increase in Type 2 diabetes, once considered an 'adults-only' disease, in children, and can lead to a variety of other weight-related medical problems later in life.

Because weight loss can be a long and bumpy road, you'll find your enthusiasm waning occasionally. Try these strategies to keep yourself inspired and on track:

· **Compete and commiserate.** Set weight-loss goals with a friend or partner. A little friendly competition can be just the motivation you need, and you'll also have someone to call to talk you down when that ice-cream sundae just won't stop calling your name.

- **Reward yourself.** Find non-edible indulgences to tell yourself 'that was a good job!'
- **Scale back.** Don't weigh yourself obsessively. Once a week – at the same time of day – is all you need to keep an eye on your progress.
- **Take baby steps.** Everyone starts somewhere. Even a walk around the block is better than sitting on the couch wishing you had the stamina to go on a bike ride with your kids.

Still need more motivation? See Chapter 12 for some alternative ways to keep exercise interesting.

What Doesn't Work

There are plenty of weight-loss strategies that are guaranteed to backfire on you:

- **Missing meals.** Foregoing food completely is hard on your diabetes control, may cause a hypo and will probably only be effective in making you eat twice as much at the next meal.
- **Missing medications.** Purposely missing your shots is spinning the DKA roulette wheel. Insulin omission is not an effective method of weight loss and can trigger dangerous highs.
- **Dieting without exercise, or vice versa.** Decreasing calories and increasing activity are both required for successful weight loss.
- **Perpetual procrastination.** Waiting for a 'better time' to start a weight-loss plan won't make it any easier, and it can quite possibly make the task harder. Stop waiting for tomorrow, and begin today.

Mind Over Matter

Losing weight with diabetes means you have two challenges to conquer: learning what and how to eat for optimal blood glucose control, and breaking away from bad overeating habits.

Eating emotionally rather than in response to hunger cues is at the root of many weight problems. Examine what your 'eating triggers' are. Do you use food as a reward, a comfort, a social tool or simply a release from boredom? The first step in breaking these habits is recognizing them and then coming up with positive substitutions.

Try to rely more on the way you feel than the tale of the tape. If the scale tells you you're losing weight slower than you'd like, but you're feeling energetic and positive about your weight-loss efforts, then you're doing fine. Again, weight loss is not a quick process.

Make a reward something that feeds your soul rather than your stomach – a few hours with a good book or a weekend getaway with someone special. Try to come up with ways to socialize that aren't focused on food. Meet at a café rather than a restaurant, or meet up to play football or Frisbee rather than spending another afternoon as an armchair centre-forward.

Above all, practise thoughtful eating. Have meals and snacks away from the television and other distractions that make it too easy to gobble up twice as much as you intended to. Enjoy your food, and then move on. Fortunately, good diabetes management encourages mindful eating.

The Low-Carbohydrate Conundrum

Low-carbohydrate diets are the subject of heated debate in the diabetes community. At first glance, the issue seems cut-and-dried. Carbohydrates cause glucose to rise, so wouldn't a low-carbohydrate diet be beneficial for someone with diabetes? But low carbohydrate also turns the traditional healthy balanced diet plate model on its head, and goes against everything that dieticians and nutritionists have been saying for decades – that the vast majority of calories (50–60 per cent) should come from carbohydrates.

In a nutshell, proponents of the low-carbohydrate diet blame weight gain on high insulin levels, which can promote fat storage. Since insulin release is triggered by dietary carbohydrates, the reasoning is that too many carbohydrates means too much glucose, which in turn leads to high levels of insulin, which cause fat storage and weight gain.

One of the most popular low-carbohydrate plans was created by the American Dr Richard Bernstein, who has Type 1 diabetes and helped to pioneer the concept of regular self-monitoring of blood glucose levels. The plan is described in his book, *Dr Bernstein's Diabetes Solution*.

The Risks Involved

The diabetes community in the UK does not endorse Atkins and similar low-carbohydrate plans, saying that the high-fat and high-protein content in these diets can be dangerous for people with diabetes who are already at risk for coronary artery disease. Also, there are a number of essential vitamins and minerals that we consume when we eat 'healthy' non-processed starchy carbohydrates, that might be lacking in a low-carbohydrate diet. Another problem with low-carb diets is that the high-protein content can be tough on the kidneys of people who have any degree of renal impairment. The Atkins Centre itself says that anyone with severe kidney disease (described as a creatinine level of 2.4 or higher) should not do the programme.

That said, there are many people who swear by them – saying that 'low-carbing' has given them their blood sugar control back. Most successful low-carbing involves attention to calories as well as carbohydrates; too much fat can add too many calories to your diet, and without calorie reduction weight loss simply won't occur. If you decide to give low-carbohydrate dieting a try, discuss it with your doctor first, and work with your dietician on a customized plan for you.

The issue of the safety of low-carb approaches was high profile enough to warrant a 2000 USDA-sponsored roundtable called 'The Great Nutrition Debate', which pitted low-carbohydrate luminaries, including the late Dr Atkins, against proponents of the diet plate and other nutritional gurus. Although the conference didn't have any far-reaching policy implications, it did reveal the growing dichotomy between the nutrition establishment and low-carbohydrate advocates.

In May 2003, the American *New England Journal of Medicine* published two controlled trials that put low-carbohydrate diets to the test among people with significant weight and health problems. One study found that obese participants with diabetes who were restricted to 30g of carbohydrates daily achieved greater weight loss, maintained better glucose control and cut triglyceride levels more than their counterparts who were put on a low-fat diet. The second trial had a smaller study population but came to similar conclusions. However, the authors also concluded that the difference in these health benefits between low fat and low carbohydrates became insignificant after the first six months. Further long-term, large-scale trials are needed to analyze the risks and potential benefits of low carbohydrates in diabetes treatment.

Glycaemic Index Diets

Then there's the glycaemic index, the subject of many bestselling diet books, such as *Sugar Busters* and *The Glucose Revolution*, and another dietary hot potato. The GI focuses on the choice of carbohydrates rather than carbohydrate restriction. Low-GI foods raise blood glucose levels at a slow and steady rate, promoting weight loss by discouraging blood glucose spikes and high circulating levels of insulin. The GI has a solid foundation in science and many faithful followers, but requires some dedicated maths skills and an even more dedicated patient. For more on the glycaemic index, see Chapter 11.

Most fad diets are just that – a fleeting fancy. At best, they drain your wallet and your self-confidence; at their worst, they can be hazardous to your health. Anything that claims dramatic results in days or a few weeks, that relies on 'testimonials' instead of hard scientific facts, or that uses lots of buzzwords to cover up a serious lack of substance is probably destined for failure.

Drugs and Surgery

When diet and exercise just aren't doing the job for whatever reason, there are other options. Some weight-loss medications, such as orlistat (marketed under the name Zenical), may have some promise in treating obesity. In clinical trials, Xenical produced a 5 per cent or higher weight loss in 72 per cent of subjects over a period of six months. The mean weight loss was 10.5kg (23lb). The National Institute for Clinical Excellence (NICE) dictate that the drug only be prescribed to people with Type 2 diabetes with a BMI > 28 if 2.5kg (6lb) in weight is lost (through diet and exercise) in the month preceding the first prescription of orlistat.

Bariatric Surgery

Finally, for severely obese people with Type 2 diabetes who have been unable to lose weight using traditional means, surgery to either reduce the size of the stomach, or to shorten the length of the digestive tract may be an option. Surgery to aid weight reduction is not commonly undertaken – in England and Wales only about 200 operations are carried out per year (and many of these are funded privately). Only patients with a BMI greater than or equal to 35 are typically considered for bariatric surgery.

There are a number of different types of bariatric surgery, including adjustable gastric banding, vertical banded gastroplasty, Roux-en-Y gastric bypass and biliopancreatic diversion (with or without a duodenal switch). The first two of these are restrictive surgeries, and work by closing off the majority of the stomach to the digestive process, leaving only a small section to digest food. The latter two are bypass (or malabsorptive) operations, which reroute the digestive flow past part or all of the small intestine to minimize the amount of calories absorbed.

Bariatric surgery carries the same risks of infection and haemorrhage as any major surgery, plus a high rate of related complications; up to 20 per cent of people who have bariatric surgery have to undergo a follow-up operation to fix abdominal hernia or other problems. Gallstones are also a risk because of the rapid weight loss that occurs following the operation.

And because some types of surgery bypass the small intestine, where a great deal of nutrient absorption takes place, approximately 30 per cent of patients end up with deficiencies of certain vitamins and minerals (a condition that can usually be corrected with supplementation).

Keeping it Off

Weight maintenance can be a lifelong challenge. Sometimes you can't control the situations that put the weight back on. Illness or injury can hamper your exercise efforts, or required drug therapy may promote weight gain. When health conditions cause weight gain, sometimes the only thing you can do is wait it out and get back on your programme when things are more settled.

Keep a diary of your weight-loss progress — it can help you become familiar with the things that trigger weight gain and slip-ups for you, and make you much less likely to fall prey to them next time around.

But slipping back into old habits like emotional eating, exercise avoidance or plain old procrastination can be avoided. In fact, having diabetes may make it easier to stay on track, since you have to pay attention to your body by default. When you do stumble, remember that it isn't the end of the world. You're simply learning another lesson about yourself and your health that will benefit your emotional management of diabetes in the long run.

Chapter 14

In Case of Emergency

One minute you're fine, the next you are dizzy, shaky and disorientated. Blood glucose highs and lows – the peaks and valleys of diabetes – are perhaps the scariest part of the disease. Preparation, prevention and patience are the keys to getting through them and staying in control of your diabetes.

Hypoglycaemic Episodes

Hypoglycaemia, also referrerd to as an insulin reaction, low blood glucose or a hypo, can hit hard and fast. If you have Type 1 diabetes, you are more likely to experience low blood glucose levels than if you have Type 2 diabetes (although people with Type 2 can experience hypos as well).

What exactly constitutes a hypo varies from person to person. Everyone has differing levels of sensitivity to blood glucose drops. One person may start to feel 'funny' at 3.9 mmol/l, while another can drop considerably lower before sensing that something is wrong. Still others suffer from a condition known as *hypoglycaemic unawareness*, in which the body no longer reacts to low blood glucose levels with the usual symptoms. Your doctor or diabetes specialist nurse will help establish what reading is too low for you.

Hypo episodes are typically caused by one of three things:

1. Too much insulin or diabetes medication (sulphonylureas or meglitinides)
2. Too little food
3. Exercise without enough carbohydrates.

Exercise naturally lowers blood glucose levels, so if you're working out, you should test before, during (about half an hour in) and after exercising. For more on exercise and diabetes, see Chapter 12.

When it comes to dealing effectively with hypoglycaemia, you need to be prepared, practise prevention and exercise patience. Carry a fast-acting sugar or carbohydrate at all times; test often and treat at the first sign of a hypo; and don't panic and down 2l of fizzy drink, or you can easily end up on a roller coaster of highs and hypos.

Signs and Symptoms

Low blood glucose levels are dangerous because the central nervous system needs glucose to function properly. That's why severe untreated hypos can cause a loss of consciousness.

Other symptoms include:
· Shakiness (trembling hands, etc.)
· Dizziness or lightheadedness
· Headache
· Hunger
· Heart palpitations
· Sudden sweating
· Clammy or pale skin
· Irritability or unexplained mood swings
· Confusion or disorientation.

Treating a Hypo

Once your blood glucose meter has confirmed a hypo, take action at once. The rule of thumb for treating low blood glucose is to take 15g of a fast-acting carbohydrate, wait 10–15 minutes, and test again. Good, quick carbohydrate options include four glucose tablets or half a glass of pure fruit juice (about 150ml). Sweets such as Smarties are also effective and portable choices. If your levels are still too low after testing the second time, have another 15g of carbohydrates. Any time you don't have your glucose monitor with you to check your blood but feel the symptoms of a hypo, trust your instincts and assume that your glucose levels are low.

Fat can delay the absorption of sugar, so if you're treating a hypo, things such as cakes, chocolate bars and ice-cream aren't the best choices. While they will do in a pinch, they will take longer to bring glucose back up. Instead, keep a packet of glucose tablets or a tube of glucose gel in your wallet or purse, car and desk, and you'll always be prepared.

It is possible to lose consciousness and/or have a seizure (a fit) when blood glucose levels drop extremely low. For this reason, it's always a good idea to have someone accessible (partner, friend, colleague, teacher) who knows exactly what to do in case of a hypoglycaemic episode.

If you are still conscious, they can assist you in taking a fast-acting carbohydrate by mouth. This should not be attempted if you are unconscious because of the risk of choking. If you lose consciousness, an injection of the hormone glucagon should be administered; if glucagon is not available, someone should call 999 immediately or transport you to the nearest Accident & Emergency hospital.

How Glucagon Works

Glucagon stimulates the liver to convert stored glycogen back into glucose. A glucagon kit contains a syringe and a vial of powdered glucagon; the fluid in the prefilled syringe is mixed with the powder immediately before use, drawn into the syringe and then injected like insulin into a large muscle like the thigh or buttock. Glucagon is available by prescription only; your doctor or diabetes specialist nurse can give you a quick lesson on how and when to use it.

Glucagon will not work to treat a hypo caused by drinking alcohol. It will also not work if there is an insufficient amount of glycogen available in the liver (such as in cases of malnutrition). Glucagon can cause nausea and possible vomiting, so you should let whoever you instruct in its use know that they should place you on your side if you are given glucagon and are still unconscious.

Always store the instructions for your glucagon injection with the syringe. Even with the best preparation, people can forget what they're supposed to be doing in an emotionally charged situation. Make sure you periodically check the expiration date on your glucagon kit, so it is always ready – just in case.

Night Hypos

Even the very idea of having a hypo in the middle of the night is frightening. Will you wake up? Will your partner wake up? If you have a child with diabetes, how will you know if she has a 2am hypo? If your blood glucose levels are below 6.0 mmol/l at bedtime, you may experience a hypo during the night. Fortunately, with a little planning and treatment adjustments, the problem is usually remedied relatively easily.

Night-time hypos are most common in people taking insulin. You pump out less glucose between midnight and 3am because your body is at rest and simply doesn't need it. If your insulin peaks during the time when glucose production is unusually low, a hypo could result.

Exercise could again be the culprit if you're working out intensely in the evening. Try a workout earlier in the day, or talk to your doctor about adjusting your insulin dose before working out to accommodate the natural drop in blood glucose that exercise produces.

A bedtime snack can often ward off middle-of-the-night drops in some people. The snack should contain protein to lengthen the release of the carbohydrate. If you are on insulin and night-time hypos persist despite treatment adjustments, an insulin pump (which can be programmed to avoid highs and lows while you sleep) may be an option.

If you're experiencing night hypos, it's a good idea to set your alarm to wake you up for several tests during the middle of the night until you've found a treatment approach that works well for you. Make sure you have glucose tablets or another quick carbohydrate on your bedside table just in case you need it. Check the testing information and review it with your doctor to try to find a pattern to your hypos.

> If you're having high morning readings, you may have to do a little detective work and set your alarm for several night-time tests in order to figure out exactly what's happening. Talk to your doctor or diabetes specialist nurse about recommendations for adjusting your insulin or treatment.

Sometimes lows that occur when you sleep cause morning fasting blood glucose levels (before breakfast) to be elevated. This phenomenon, known as the *Somogyi effect* or *rebound*, happens when the body starts producing glucagon and adrenaline in response to a hypo. These hormones signal the liver to convert glycogen to glucose, and the result is high blood glucose levels upon waking. If your blood glucose is high at your first morning test, there's a possibility it's due to an undetected night-time hypo. However, it may also be a result of the *dawn phenomenon*, which is a morning high caused by the natural release of blood glucose in the early-morning hours.

Hypoglycaemic Unawareness

Sometimes people who have had diabetes for many years develop hypoglycaemic unawareness – blood glucose lows that you don't know about because you don't experience any symptoms. This may be caused in part by damage to the sympathetic nervous system (called autonomic neuropathy), in which the typical involuntary reactions to low blood glucose levels – such as sweating and flushes – don't occur. For some people with this condition, a loss of consciousness is their first and only sign that their blood glucose has dipped dangerously low.

Another situation that can trigger hypoglycaemic unawareness in some patients is a regime of intensive or tight blood glucose control. These patients are three times more likely to experience hypoglycaemic unawareness than those on a non-intensive treatment programme. If you have a hypo, your risk of having yet another one is higher for up to two days following the episode. If you're trying to keep your blood glucose levels in tight control, you have a fine line to walk, and it's possible to end up in a vicious cycle of hypo after hypo. Eventually, hypoglycaemic unawareness may result.

f@ct

Several studies have found that moderate intake of caffeine may be useful in heightening sensitivity to symptoms of blood glucose hypos in those patients with hypoglycaemic unawareness. Be sure to check with your doctor first, as too much caffeine can have negative consequences, particularly if you have high blood pressure.

If you develop hypoglycaemic unawareness while on an intensive control programme, your doctor will probably recommend increasing your target blood glucose levels slightly to avoid dangerous lows. Some clinical studies have shown that loosening control to allow blood glucose levels to run slightly high for two to three weeks can restore hypoglycaemia awareness in some patients. Blood glucose awareness training may also be an option for you if you have hypoglycaemic unawareness. Frequent monitoring, paying increased attention to hypo triggers, and recognition of some of the subtler signs of a hypo are the focus of this training.

Can the GlucoWatch help stop lows at night?

The GlucoWatch Biographer (Cygnus), a continuous blood monitoring system, can detect episodes of hypoglycaemia, and several studies have demonstrated that it can reduce the incidence of night-time hypoglycaemic episodes in children. However, you should always follow up any low glucose alarms with a regular finger stick glucose test, as the GlucoWatch can give false positive readings.

Anyone who experiences blood glucose readings of 2.5 mmol/l or less without any signs of hypoglycaemia should inform their doctor promptly.

Diabetic Ketoacidosis (DKA)

On the other end of the spectrum is hyperglycaemia, or high blood glucose. If glucose levels reach 13.9 mmol/l or higher and ketones are present in the blood or urine, these may be indications that diabetic ketoacidosis (DKA) has occurred.

DKA is most common in Type 1 diabetes, although it can also occur in people with Type 2. It happens when, in the absolute or relative deficiency of insulin (which enables the body to use glucose for energy), the body starts to break down fat for energy instead. Fat metabolism causes ketone bodies to form, throwing the acid balance off-kilter in the bloodstream. Meanwhile, the liver continues to pump out more and more glucose in a fruitless attempt to fuel the body, and blood glucose climbs higher and higher. The result is ketoacidosis.

When the body is under a severe degree of stress, hyperglycaemia and possible DKA are a danger. Infection, injury, surgical procedures and even a simple cold or flu are all known offenders in causing blood glucose to rise. Sometimes people miss their insulin or medication because they are ill, which boosts blood glucose even higher. Dehydration caused by vomiting and diarrhoea can also worsen blood glucose levels.

Eating disorders can also be an underlying cause of DKA, particularly in adolescents with Type 1 diabetes. One American study of women with Type 1 found that 31 per cent intentionally missed an insulin dose at some point, while 8.8 per cent of those did it regularly. Reasons given for omitting insulin treatment included fear of weight gain and fear of hypoglycaemia. The researchers also hypothesized that emotional issues related to living with chronic diabetes could be a cause of omission.

Never skip a dose of insulin or diabetes medication just because you are ill – even if you're not eating much. Illness usually causes blood glucose levels to climb, and missing medication can make the problem worse. In many cases, you may require more insulin when you are ill. Talk to your doctor about a 'sick day plan' for your medications and/or insulin dose.

Signs and Symptoms

Often the symptoms of DKA are ignored initially because many closely resemble the flu or a viral infection. The fact that the flu itself causes blood glucose levels to rise and can trigger DKA complicates matters further. This is why frequent testing and staying on your treatment schedule are so important when you are ill. Symptoms of DKA include:

- Fruity smell on the breath (from acetone)
- Nausea
- Vomiting
- Fatigue
- Muscle aches and stiffness
- Abdominal pain
- Extreme thirst and frequent urination
- Rapid breathing or difficulty breathing
- Mental confusion
- Unconsciousness or, in extreme cases, coma.

A rare but potentially fatal complication of DKA, cerebral oedema (swelling of the brain), is a particular risk in children. Signs of cerebral oedema include severe headache, irritability, drowsiness and confusion.

Treating DKA

Diabetic ketoacidosis should always be treated in a hospital setting. Treatment consists of lowering blood glucose levels with insulin and restoring fluid and electrolyte balance with intravenous saline. In some cases, potassium or other electrolytes may also be administered intravenously. If the underlying cause of the DKA is illness or infection, it should be treated appropriately to prevent recurrence.

When to Test for Ketones

If your blood glucose levels are 14.0 mmol/l or higher, you should test for ketones. Ketone testing is particularly important when you are ill, and during pregnancy. Ketones can be picked up in the urine by a simple test using a chemically teated reagent strip (see Chapter 6). There is also a combination blood glucose and ketone meter (MediSense Optium) available that is useful for home testing. Blood testing for ketones is superior to urine testing, and should be done preferentially.

Hyperosmolar Nonketotic Coma (HONK)

Another complication of extremely high blood glucose levels, hyperosmolar hyperglycaemia (also called hyperosmolar nonketotic coma, or HONK) occurs most frequently in patients with Type 2 diabetes. In HONK, hyperglycaemia occurs without ketosis (the formation of ketone bodies). Extreme dehydration results in a dangerous drop in blood pressure and potential cardiovascular collapse. For this reason, there is a high mortality rate with HONK.

fact

Certain medications that raise blood glucose levels, such as steroids, atypical antipsychotics, glucocorticoids and diuretics, can cause dangerous hyperglycaemic episodes.

Often, people who develop HONK are on drugs that raise their blood glucose levels, or become dehydrated due to diuretic medications or illness. The condition occurs commonly in elderly patients with previously undiagnosed diabetes. Having impaired kidney function also increases your risk of developing HONK.

HONK can occur at blood glucose levels of about 30 mmol/l. At diagnosis, plasma glucose is usually much higher than in DKA (around 55 mmol/l).

Signs and Symptoms

As opposed to DKA, which usually has a rapid onset, HONK may be subtler, taking days to weeks to build up to a crisis point. If you are ill and your glucose levels are persistently above 14 mmol/l, even if you test negative for ketones, you should still call your doctor for further advice. If you exhibit any of the signs of HONK along with high blood glucose levels, you should call your doctor immediately or go to the nearest Accident & Emergency facility.

Possible symptoms of HONK include:

·   Frequent urination
·   Excessive thirst
·   Nausea and vomiting
·   Weight loss
·   Dehydration
·   Weakness
·   Seizures
·   Confusion, unconsciousness or coma.

Treating HONK

Treatment for HONK is similar to that for diabetic ketoacidosis. Restoring the fluid balance to the bloodstream is the immediate goal. A saline solution is administered via an intravenous drip, and electrolytes may also be administered. Insulin therapy may or may not be needed. Finding out the root cause or event that precipitated the HONK is key in preventing its recurrence. HONK has a significantly higher fatality rate, and must always be treated in hospital.

High-Risk Situations

There are several situations that cause blood glucose levels to nosedive or skyrocket. Being prepared for them when and if they occur is the best way to avoid the potential highs and lows.

Sick Days

Being ill is a big risk factor for high blood glucose levels. If your doctor hasn't discussed it with you already, you should ask him about developing a 'sick day plan', which is simply a course of action to take if you develop flu or another mild illness. Here are some guidelines to follow when you are ill:

- **Keep eating and drinking.** Have plenty of food and drinks on hand that are easy on the stomach, including soup and sandwiches, toast or crackers, milk and biscuits, or mashed banana with yoghurt. Drink plenty of water and fluids to avoid dehydration.
- **Stock up the medicine cabinet.** In addition to your glucose meter, you should always have ketone-testing supplies on hand, plus basics such as a thermometer and medications to treat diarrhoea and vomiting. Talk to your doctor about recommendations for the latter.
- **Stay in touch.** Discuss guidelines with your doctor or diabetes specialist nurse about when you should call (e.g. if your blood glucose reaches a certain landmark, if you can't keep food down, or if you exhibit specific symptoms). When in doubt, always pick up the phone.

- **Test often.** Stating the obvious – you'll need to test frequently to pick up dangerous highs early.
- **Don't miss your medication.** Keep taking both insulin and oral medications, even if you aren't eating very much, and if they aren't bringing down your glucose adequately, call your doctor to discuss increasing the dose.

> **tips**
>
> Diabetes UK recommend that people with diabetes follow the principles of sensible drinking: two units per day if you are a woman, or three units per day if you are a man. It takes the body up to two hours to metabolize, or clear, 2ml of alcohol from the body, so test frequently after you drink.

Drinking Alcohol

When you drink, your liver shuts down its regular glycogen storage and glucose production operation. The result can be hypoglycaemia, either while you're drinking or hours afterwards, while your liver continues to clear alcohol from the bloodstream. For this reason, you should always eat when you drink, and be on the lookout for symptoms of a hypo.

If you choose to drink alcohol, it is absolutely essential that you have a non-drinking friend with you who knows how to recognize the symptoms of hypoglycaemia and treat them appropriately. Because alcohol can so easily impair judgment, this should be a person you can trust not to drink.

Always eat something when you drink, to keep glucose levels up, and be sure to assess any mixed drinks for 'hidden' calories and sugar from fruit juices or mixes (and work them into your overall meal plan). A snack before bed is also important if you've indulged, to ward off overnight hyops. It's always a good idea to set your alarm to awaken you for a middle of the night blood test for the same reason.

Even if you choose to abstain or have only one drink, but attend a function where the alcohol is flowing freely, it's important to have a designated (non)drinking friend who knows what to look out for. Some of the symptoms of a hypo – confusion, mood swings and incoherence –

can easily be mistaken for intoxication by others (especially if they've had a few themselves) and not treated appropriately.

Medications

Certain medications can cause highs or lows. Whenever you get a new prescription, ask your doctor about its potential of affecting your blood glucose levels and what adjustments you can make to your treatment to avoid an emergency situation. For the same reason, never take supplements or herbal remedies without discussing them with your doctor first.

Make sure you are never caught without your diabetes medication. Always make sure to get your insulin and oral drug prescriptions well before you run out.

Support System

Embarrassed, ashamed, self-conscious, guilty, alone – do any of these describe the way you're feeling about having diabetes? First of all, realize that you aren't to blame for having this disease. These feelings are a natural part of coming to terms with your diagnosis. It may take some time to overcome them completely, but in the meantime you need to get past them enough to let the people around you know you need their help.

At the time of writing this book, there were over 1.4 million people living with diabetes in the UK. That makes the odds pretty good that at least a few of your colleagues, neighbours, friends and family have already been touched by the disease on some level. With that in mind, you may not need to tell them a lot they don't already know; then again, they may be badly in need of some accurate and current diabetes education. Either way, you only have to share the basics of handling an emergency at this point.

First off, have a 'diabetes friend' (or two or three) at each place you frequent regularly, such as work, the gym or playing field, class, work etc. Let them know (and give them access to) where you keep your basic supplies (i.e.,meter, fast-acting glucose, glucagon kit) and provide them with instructions on administering glucagon. Most of the glucagon kits on the market have illustrated instructions with them that make giving an injection easier.

When educating friends, family and colleagues about emergency situations, make sure they understand the difference between insulin and glucagon. Since both are injected, they may easily be confused, a situation that could have life-threatening consequences if you were to lose consciousness and were treated with the wrong drug.

These basic guidelines can give your support team directions for offering you assistance. You can customize them to your own particular blood glucose numbers:

· If I look ill or am acting strange, ask me if I'm OK and suggest that I check my blood glucose levels.
· If I test low (under 4 mmol/l or as indicated by a low alarm on my meter) and am still conscious, help me to eat or drink some glucose tablets, juice or other fast-acting sugars.
· If I test extremely high (over 14 mmol/l or as indicated by a high alarm on my meter) and I lose consciousness or am incoherent, call 999 or get me to A&E immediately.
· If I test low and lose consciousness, do not try to feed me. Call 999 immediately and administer a glucagon injection.
· If I haven't tested or you don't know what my blood glucose levels were and I lose consciousness, never try to feed me or give me insulin or glucagon. Instead, call 999 immediately.

Medical Identification

Even if you've got a friend with you at all times, it's important to make sure that you have medical identification in case you need to be treated by medical personnel. You don't need to sport a giant scarlet *D* on your lapel, but wearing some form of ID at all times is the best way to ensure that you will get proper treatment should a blood glucose emergency cause you to lose consciousness among strangers.

It may be tempting to take off your ID at the gym or before a run. Don't. During (and following) exercise is a high-risk time for hypoglycaemia. The same goes for social events and parties with alcohol. Living with diabetes means that blood glucose lows and highs can strike at any time. Don't be caught unprepared.

The Options

When you're shopping for medical ID, keep these elements in mind:

- It must be noticeable – the most important criterion for a good ID.
- It must be comfortable – otherwise you won't wear it.
- It should be durable enough to stand up to sun, surf and whatever other elements you may encounter.
- It should be comprehensive – make sure it lists all your pertinent medical information.
- It should be stylish. Make sure you like it, or, again, you won't wear it.

Your ID should indicate that you have diabetes. If you take insulin, it should say that as well, along with any drug allergies you may have. Your tag will let paramedics and other health care providers know that they should test your blood glucose before treating you.

What Works and What Doesn't

Some people don't like to shout out 'I have diabetes!' and opt for less intrusive means of identification, such as a key chain or a wallet card. Unfortunately, being subtle doesn't do you much good in an emergency situation. If you collapse, probably the only person who would go immediately for your wallet or your car keys would be a mugger or car thief. A medical alert bracelet, pendant or watchband is much more likely to be noticed for the right reasons.

Make it a habit to always test your blood glucose before you drive. If it's too low, treat it and wait for the subsequent rise before turning on the ignition. Even the slightest lapse in concentration can have serious repercussions behind the wheel of a car. Driving with low blood glucose levels can be just as dangerous as drinking and driving.

Many medical IDs are marked with a caduceus – a winged staff entwined with snakes that is the Greek symbol for medicine. Today's medical ID products are available in a wide variety of configurations, including watch tags, bracelets, pendants, sports bands, shoelace tags, clip-on ID cards, custom-made gemstone jewellery and even temporary tattoos. Products such as shoelace tags (which are worn securely at the toe end of the laces) are good choices for young children who may not like to wear bracelets or pendants.

Emergency Response Services

If you have a complicated medical history, or simply want to have more peace of mind regarding treatment of your diabetes in an emergency, you can invest in a subscription to an emergency response service. These companies store your detailed medical information in a database, then issue you medical identification engraved with both your medical condition and their number (often a free-phone one). When hospital or emergency personnel call the number, your information can be relayed to them. If you aren't willing or able to make an investment in this type of service, some standard ID products feature compartments for storing more extensive written medical information.

Chapter 15

Complications –
Head to Toe

Your body is equipped with 96,000km (60,000 miles) of blood vessels and wired with a whopping 160,000km (100,000 miles) of nerve fibres. A block here, some corrosion there, and all this hardware suffers from the strain. Diabetes is like a bad tenant, backing up pipes and short-circuiting wiring. You may not be able to evict it, but you can do your part to prevent long-term systemic complications with proper maintenance.

Neurological Complications

Diabetes is a risk factor for strokes, nerve damage and cognitive impairment. While a stroke is technically a cardiovascular complication caused by a blockage of blood to or a haemorrhage in the brain, it can cause impairment to memory, vision, speech, movement and other brain functions in varying degrees of severity.

The other major neurological complications of diabetes are caused by neuropathy, or nerve damage. The exact way in which diabetes causes nerve damage is not completely understood yet, but it's thought that over a period of time, high levels of blood glucose damage the nerve cells, which, unlike other cells, don't require an insulin 'key' to allow glucose inside them. Researchers also hypothesize that too much glucose causes depletion of nitric acid, which in turn cuts off blood supply to the nerves.

Neuropathies are either *diffuse* (affecting a wide area or several areas of the body) or *focal* (affecting a specific place on the body). Most neuropathic conditions related to diabetes are diffuse, including peripheral and autonomic neuropathy.

Peripheral Neuropathy (PN)

Peripheral neuropathy most commonly affects the feet and hands. The condition can be particularly troublesome in the feet because of the chance that you may develop an injury that you don't notice, and compound the problem through the simple act of walking (for more on PN and your feet, see Chapter 16).

Symptoms of peripheral neuropathy include:

·   A feeling of pins and needles
·   Tingling and/or burning sensations
·   In some people, pain
·   Numbness
·   Balance problems (if PN is present in the feet)
·   Reflex problems and muscle weakness.

Antidepressant medications (amitriptyline and nortriptyline) may be useful in blocking pain signals, although side effects may be an issue for some patients. The anticonvulsant drug gabapentin (Neurontin) is an effective treatment for many people with PN and has the additional advantage of having few side effects. A number of studies have also shown promising treatment results with alpha lipoic acid (ALA) treatment, although ALA is not approved for use at this point in time.

Over half of men over the age of 50 with diabetes have impotence problems, which can be related to both neuropathy and cardiovascular complications. In women, diabetes can affect oestrogen levels, menstrual and ovulation cycles and sexual desire.

Treatment with capsaicin cream (Axsain or Zacin), which contains a substance derived from hot peppers that helps to block pain signals, may also be recommended by your doctor. And some anecdotal success has been reported in treating PN with acupuncture and with transcutaneous electronic nerve stimulations (TENS), which uses electricity to block pain signals.

Autonomic Neuropathy

While many people with diabetes are aware of the signs and symptoms of PN, significantly fewer are educated about, or tested for, autonomic neuropathy. A stealth disorder, autonomic neuropathy short-circuits the nerves that control the sympathetic (autonomic, or involuntary) nervous system. Blood pressure, heart rate, perspiration, salivation, gastrointestinal and bladder function, sexual potency and vision can all be impaired by autonomic neuropathy.

Autonomic neuropathy causes a wide spectrum of non-specific symptoms, ranging from constipation and diarrhoea to dizziness and excessive perspiration (see overleaf). Unfortunately, these are also common signs of a number of medical conditions, which makes autonomic neuropathy particularly difficult to detect without regular screening. Sometimes, a diagnosis isn't made until organ damage has occurred.

Autonomic Neuropathy		
	Symptoms	**Possible Associated Complications**

Cardiovascular system	Dizziness
	Drop in blood pressure
	Less variation than normal in
	  heart rate
	Elevated resting heart rate
	Shortness of breath
	Perspiration
		Orthostatic hypotension
		Silent heart attack
		Serious heart rhythm
		  abnormalities

Digestive system	Constipation Diarrhoea Bloating and nausea Premature feeling of fullness	Gastroparesis
Genito-urinary	Urinary tract infections Urinary incontinence Vaginal dryness Inability to maintain erection Decreased or increased urination	Neurogenic bladder Impotence
Sudomotor system	Increased perspiration (trunk and face) Decreased perspiration (extremities) Dry, thick skin on hands and feet	Skin rashes and infection
Vision	Small pupils No pupil response to light/dark	Impaired night vision

Cardiovascular Autonomic Neuropathy (CAN)

This disorder begins silently without symptoms of chest pain or discomfort (angina), and often remains undetected until serious myocardial infarction (death of the heart muscle due to lack of oxygen) has occurred. As a result, these 'silent heart attacks' often pass without proper medical attention.

If you experience any unexplained shortness of breath, weakness and fatigue and/or excessive perspiration – all possible symptoms of silent heart attack – report it to your doctor promptly. The mortality rate of CAN is up to 50 per cent within five years once symptoms appear, so early diagnosis is essential.

I get dizzy when I stand up suddenly, and my doctor said it could be neuropathy. Isn't that a foot condition?

Your doctor is talking about autonomic neuropathy. Cardiovascular autonomic neuropathy can trigger a sudden drop in blood pressure known as orthostatic (postural) hypotension. When you stand up, blood vessel and nerve damage prevent your blood pressure from rising quickly enough to compensate for the change in position, and dizziness, vision problems and lightheadedness result.

Patients with CAN have little variation in their heart rate, which typically remains continuously elevated both at rest and under stress (e.g. after exercise). Heart rate variability (HRV) testing is used to diagnose the condition. HRV testing involves assessing the heart rate during activities of deep breathing, a postural test (i.e. lying down, rising and standing), and the Valsalva manoeuvre. The Valsalva manoeuvre is performed by bearing down, or forcefully breathing out through the mouth with both the mouth and nose closed. In patients without CAN, the heart rate should slow during this manoeuvre. If the heart rate remains consistent (i.e. does not slow or speed up) during all three of these activities, CAN is suspected.

Autonomic neuropathy can also cause hypoglycaemic unawareness, a potentially serious inability to detect the physical symptoms of a low blood glucose episode.

Cognitive Impairment

People with diabetes may experience memory problems and cognitive impairment, but it isn't completely clear whether these problems are a result of physical processes, the social and psychological toll of the disease, or a combination of the two.

There is some evidence that impaired glucose tolerance, a precursor to Type 2 diabetes, can cause memory loss and atrophy of the hippocampus (the part of the brain responsible for learning and memory). Research has also indicated a greater risk for cognitive impairment in people with Type 1 diabetes, possibly because of their increased risk and incidence of hypoglycaemia.

There are plenty of medical reasons for children and their parents to avoid hypoglycaemia, of course, but researchers disagree on whether long-term cognitive dysfunction is one of them. Some studies have shown a connection between severe hypoglycaemia and learning difficulties in children with Type 1 diabetes, but others have contradicted this finding.

Musculoskeletal Complications

In addition to peripheral neuropathy, there are several other complications of diabetes that affect the musculoskeletal system and the extremities.

Frozen Shoulder

Frozen shoulder, or adhesive capsulitis, is a disorder of the connective tissue that limits the normal range of motion of the shoulder. In diabetes, it is caused by changes to the collagen in the shoulder joint as a result of long-term hyperglycaemia. It usually happens in one shoulder only, although it can occur in both.

Physiotherapy focused on improving the range of motion, along with anti-inflammatory medications, is usually the first line of treatment for frozen shoulder. Cortisone injections are also sometimes used in the treatment of frozen shoulder.

Conditions involving inflammation of the tendons or joints are sometimes treated with non-steroidal anti-inflammatory medications (NSAIDs) such as ibuprofen. However, NSAIDs should be prescribed with care in patients with kidney disease and/or cardiovascular disease, as they have the potential to worsen these conditions.

Dupuytren's Contracture

Another condition that limits range of motion is Dupuytren's contracture. As its common name, trigger finger, suggests, the condition is characterized by pain, stiffness and a 'locking' of the index finger. The tendon in the finger becomes inflamed and the tendon sheath, or covering, is damaged. Flexing the finger becomes increasingly difficult, and eventually the finger may lock up in a 'trigger pull' position. Again, anti-inflammatories and physiotherapy may be prescribed. In some cases, surgery may be required to correct the condition.

Carpal Tunnel Syndrome

Often confused with or mistaken for peripheral neuropathy, carpal tunnel syndrome involves nerve entrapment rather than nerve damage. The medial nerve (a nerve that runs through your wrist) becomes compressed, or entrapped, in the ligaments that surround it (the carpal tunnel). This can be caused by repetitive stress (such as that caused by typing or playing guitar), and is exacerbated by diabetes because high blood glucose can cause changes to the collagen in the ligaments, making entrapment more likely.

The result is tingling, pins and needles and burning sensations similar to what you might feel in PN. In fact, your doctor may refer to it as a *compression neuropathy* because it causes these symptoms. The difference is that carpal tunnel usually affects just the first three fingers of the hand (thumb, index and middle fingers; although sometimes the half of the ring finger closest to the middle finger is involved), while PN involves the entire hand.

Carpal tunnel syndrome is treated with wrist splints and sometimes corticosteroid injections. In some cases, surgery may be required to relieve pressure on the medial nerve.

What is stiff-hand syndrome, and how can I treat it?
Stiff-hand syndrome (digital sclerosis) is caused by a build-up of collagen under the skin. It generally doesn't cause any pain, but it can affect your flexibility. Talk to your doctor or physiotherapist about a regime of hand-stretching exercises that may help relieve the stiffness. Paraffin wax is also used as a treatment sometimes, but should only be applied by a health care professional because of the risk of burns.

Cardiovascular Complications

According to Diabetes UK, more than 20,000 people with diabetes in the UK die from coronary heart disease (CHD) every year – that's 15 per cent of all deaths from CHD. Having diabetes increases your risk of heart disease and stroke two to four times. That's a huge effect, yet few people with diabetes are aware of their increased cardiovascular risks.

Bringing blood glucose, blood pressure and LDL cholesterol levels down is the best way to combat diabetes-related cardiovascular complications. This means tightening up on blood glucose control, stopping smoking, becoming active and making appropriate dietary adjustments, such as reducing your intake of saturated fat. If, despite your best efforts, your cholesterol levels remain high (total cholesterol over 5 mmol/l and/or LDL cholesterol > 3 mmol/l), then a drug called a statin – such as atorvastatin (Lipitor), pravastatin (Lipostat) or simvastatin (Zocor) – may be prescribed.

For patients with a poor cholesterol profile, dietary adjustments (i.e. lowering intake of saturated fat) and increased exercise are recommended. If these don't provide sufficient improvement, or if LDL and/or triglyceride levels are significantly elevated to begin with, drugs called statins – such as Lipitor (atorvastatin), Pravachol (pravastatin) or Zocor (simvastatin) – may be prescribed.

Atherosclerosis and CAD

Atherosclerosis, more commonly known as hardening or clogging of the arteries, is caused by a build-up of fatty material (also called plaque or cholesterol), which restricts blood flow. For patients with arterial obstructions, medications such as nitroglycerin, beta-blockers and angiotensin-converting enzyme (ACE) inhibitors may be prescribed.

Blockage to the arteries that feed the heart is called coronary artery disease (CAD). What makes CAD particularly dangerous is that symptoms don't typically appear until vessels are significantly blocked. Symptoms of CAD include:

·   Chest pain (angina)
·   Pain in the left arm or shoulder (referred pain)
·   Neck or jaw pain
·   Chest tightness or pressure
·   Shortness of breath
·   Nausea
·   Perspiration
·   Irregular heartbeat (arrhythmia).

An electrocardiogram (ECG), echocardiogram and/or stress test may be helpful in diagnosing blocked arteries. If CAD is left untreated, the artery may become completely blocked. When blood flow is severely restricted to the heart or completely blocked off, myocardial infarction (heart attack) occurs. Without oxygen from the blood, the affected area of heart muscle dies. Symptoms of a heart attack are the same as those described previously for CAD, except that the pain is considerably more intense, and the symptoms prolonged. However, in people with diabetes who suffer from autonomic neuropathy, pain symptoms may not be felt at all, resulting in a 'silent heart attack'.

In cases of stroke or heart attack, where restoring blood flow is critical to prevent tissue death and damage, clot-dissolving or 'clot-busting' (fibrinolytic or thrombolytic) drugs may be administered – such as altepase (Actilyse), streptokinase (Streptase), reteplase (Rapilysin) or tenecteplase (Metalyse).

In those at risk, an aspirin a day may keep heart disease at bay. Diabetes UK recommends that people with diabetes over the age of 30, in high-risk groups, should be offered aspirin treatment, or should obtain it for themselves, in addition to following a healthy lifestyle. The recommended dosage is at least 75mg. Ask your doctor if you think you might benefit from taking a daily dose of aspirin. Aspirin therapy is not recommended for those with aspirin allergy, uncontrolled high blood pressure, liver problems or bleeding disorders, or if taking an anticoagulant therapy (warfarin).

You may also require an angioplasty, a procedure in which a catheter is inserted into the artery and an attached balloon is expanded to clear the blockage. Sometimes, a device called a stent, which is expanded inside the artery to hold the vessel open, is used. Atherectomy, a procedure that strips fatty blockages out of the artery, may also be performed.

Studies have indicated that coronary bypass surgery may have better long-term outcomes than angioplasty for people with diabetes. Bypass involves rerouting the circulation by grafting a healthy piece of artery onto the obstructed blood vessel and around the blockage.

Peripheral Vascular Disease (PVD)

Like CAD, peripheral vascular disease (also called peripheral arterial disease, or PAD) involves atherosclerosis. Unlike CAD, PVD affects the extremities – most commonly the legs. Signs of PVD include:

· Calf and leg cramp, usually when walking (intermittent claudication)
· Smooth, shiny, hairless skin on the shins
· Chronically cold feet and legs
· Numb legs or feet
· A bluish or reddish cast to the skin of the feet and/or legs
· Sores or ulcers on the legs that won't heal.

The treatment of PVD is similar to that of CAD. Weight loss, cholesterol improvement through diet or drug therapy, appropriate exercise and medication may all be recommended. Good foot care, important for everyone with diabetes, is especially essential for people who develop PVD.

Congestive heart failure (CHF) is yet another cardiovascular condition that people with diabetes are at a higher risk of developing. Symptoms include fluid retention (oedema), shortness of breath, heart palpitations, fatigue and low tolerance for exercise. CHF is usually treated with ACE inhibitors, digoxin and diuretics. In some cases, beta-blockers may also be prescribed.

Hypertension

Another leading complication on the diabetes hit parade is hypertension, or high blood pressure. It occurs in up to 65 per cent of people with diabetes, and is also closely linked with both diabetic kidney disease and CAD, making it a complex yet critical-to-manage condition.

Diabetes UK recommends that anyone with a blood pressure greater than 140/80 mmHg (more commonly referred to simply as '140 over 80') should receive treatment. However, stricter targets are frequently cited for people with existing diabetic complications, especially the early signs of kidney disease.

If lifestyle modifications don't bring down your blood pressure, medications such as angiotensin-converting enzyme (ACE) inhibitors, beta-blockers, diuretics and angiotensin receptor blockers (ARBs) are effective options for some people. ACE inhibitors have been shown to have the added benefit of delaying the progression of kidney disease, and may be a preferred therapy for patients who also have renal impairment. Your doctor can tell you more about these drugs and whether they may be right for you.

Stroke

Another potential cardiovascular complication of diabetes is ischaemic stroke. Ischaemic stroke occurs when an artery leading to the brain becomes blocked and blood flow is cut off. Symptoms of stroke hit suddenly and include the following:

· Weakness or numbness of the arm, face or leg (usually one-sided)
· Mental confusion
· Difficulty speaking
· Dizziness and/or problems with balance
· Visual problems
· Severe headache.

If you have diabetes, you are at higher risk for a transient ischaemic attack (TIA, or ministroke). A ministroke is characterized by the typical symptoms of stroke, but it resolves on its own without treatment. If you think you've had a ministroke, tell your doctor immediately. It is a warning sign that something is wrong, and you are at risk for a full-blown stroke.

Because of the complex relationships between diabetes and all the systems of the body, many diabetic complications are interrelated. For example, University of Wisconsin research (the Atherosclerosis Risk in Communities Study) in the USA found that middle-aged people who had never experienced a stroke but suffered from eye disease (retinopathy) displayed poorer cognitive function than those who didn't have retinopathy. The finding suggests that cerebral microvascular disease (which is at the root of diabetic retinopathy) may contribute to the development of cognitive impairment, even when stroke doesn't occur.

Visual Complications

The longer you have had diabetes, the greater your risk for visual complications from the disease. Nearly everyone who has Type 1 diabetes, and the majority of those with Type 2 diabetes, will experience some degree of retinopathy in their lifetime. The good news is that early diagnosis and treatment with laser surgery can prevent serious vision loss in the majority of cases.

Retinopathy

Diabetic retinopathy is the primary cause of new-onset blindness in people of working age. The condition is caused by blockage and/or leaking of the blood vessels that feed the retina of the eye. Swelling of the macula, part of the retina, is called macular oedema, and is a possible complication that can cause blurred vision. Often, symptoms of retinopathy are not noticed until they reach an advanced, or proliferative, stage.

Laser treatment is usually recommended for treating diabetic retinopathy. Depending on the progression of the disease, lasers may be used to either seal leaky blood vessels or destroy abnormal vessels completely.

A vitrectomy, a surgical procedure that replaces the vitreous fluid of the eye with a clear saline solution, may also be performed if blood vessels have haemorrhaged significantly into the vitreous. Both laser treatment and vitrectomy are usually hospital outpatient procedures that are performed by an ophthalmologist or eye surgeon.

tips

You need a dilated eye examination at least annually to detect diabetic eye disease early. Other essentials for good eye health include stopping the smoking habit, lowering blood pressure and keeping your HbA1c down. The Diabetes Control and Complications Trial (DCCT) found that people with uncontrolled blood glucose levels developed retinopathy four times more frequently than those who practised tight blood glucose control.

Glaucoma

Glaucoma is caused by pressure build-up in the eye that can damage the optic nerve. In cases where the normal drainage patterns of the eye are blocked, the aqueous fluids of the eye build up and put pressure on the optic nerve. A loss of peripheral (side) vision is often the first sign of glaucoma. Depending on the type of glaucoma, you may also experience severe headaches. The condition may be treated with special eye drops that lower the pressure level in the eyes. Laser surgery may also be recommended for glaucoma.

Cataracts

People with diabetes are more likely to develop cataracts at an earlier age than the general population. If you have diabetes, you are also twice as likely to develop the condition. Cataracts are characterized by a clouding of the lens of the eye. Symptoms include cloudy or fuzzy vision, double vision and sensitivity to bright light.

Mild cataracts may not require surgical intervention, unless vision is significantly reduced. Surgical treatment involves removing the clouded, natural lens and replacing it with a plastic lens that has been calibrated for your vision needs. The prognosis is excellent for anyone undergoing cataract surgery, and the procedure improves vision in an estimated 95 per cent of cases. However, there are some risks for people who also have diabetic retinopathy, as lens replacement can cause a worsening of that condition. Your doctor can provide you with information on the risks and benefits of cataract surgery in your specific medical situation.

Kidney Disease

Your kidneys are two of the hardest-working organs in your body, filtering approximately 185l of fluid from the blood that passes through them daily. After the million or so nephrons in each kidney balance electrolytes and filter toxins, around 183l of fluid are returned to the bloodstream cleansed and chemically and hormonally balanced. The remaining couple of litres leave the body as urine.

Blood vessel damage and hypertension associated with diabetes can take a serious toll on renal (or kidney) function, damaging this amazing filtration capacity of the kidneys. As a result, diabetes has become the number one cause of end-stage renal disease (ESRD, or chronic kidney failure), accounting for 35 per cent of all cases.

Both Type 1 and Type 2 diabetes patients are at risk of developing kidney problems, and the risk of developing ESRD increases with the length of time since diabetes diagnosis, possibly due to the prevalence of high blood pressure in diabetes and the added stress that this places on the kidneys.

Signs and symptoms of kidney disease include the following:

· Blood and/or protein (albumin) in the urine
· High blood pressure
· Frequent urination, especially at night
· Leg cramps
· Puffiness and swelling around the eyes, hands and feet (oedema)
· Excessive itching (pruritis)
· Nausea and vomiting
· Weakness.

If your doctor suspects that there may be renal impairment, she will run several diagnostic tests to assess your kidney function, including a urine test for microalbumin, or trace amounts of protein in the urine.

Microalbuminuria is one of the hallmarks of early kidney disease, and at one time was thought to be the beginning of the end of kidney function for people with diabetes. However, a Joslin Diabetes Centre study published in the American *New England Journal of Medicine* in June 2003 found that 58 per cent of Type 1 study subjects who developed microalbuminuria were actually able to reverse the condition within six years with good control of blood glucose, blood pressure and cholesterol levels.

Importance of Good Control

Several large-scale diabetes studies have demonstrated that tight blood glucose control can significantly reduce the risk of nephropathy. In fact, the DCCT found that people with Type 1 diabetes who maintained an average HbA1c of 7.2 per cent cut their risk of developing nephropathy and other complications up to 75 per cent. The United Kingdom Prospective Diabetes Study (UKPDS) found that people with Type 2 diabetes achieved a 35 per cent reduction in risk for nephropathy for each percentage point they lowered their A1c levels.

If you develop kidney disease, you may have to watch your protein intake; your dietician can help you to develop a meal plan that is lower in dietary protein and compatible with blood sugar control goals, if necessary. However, studies are still inconclusive on the benefits of low-protein diets in lowering the risk of developing kidney disease, and Diabetes UK currently says that with the lack of conclusive evidence, it is inappropriate to issue any general recommendation about protein intake for people with diabetic nephropathy.

Because diabetic kidney disease often goes hand in hand with hypertension, you may be prescribed ACE inhibitors or other medication to control your blood pressure, and in addition to cut the workload of your kidneys.

Kidney failure is an irreversible condition. Once kidney function diminishes to less than 10 to 15 per cent and ESRD occurs, haemodialysis, peritoneal dialysis or kidney transplant are the only treatment options.

Digestive Complications

Gastroparesis, or delayed stomach emptying, literally means partial stomach paralysis. It is another type of autonomic neuropathy caused by damage to the vagus nerve, which is responsible for facilitating the passage of food through the digestive system. What makes gastroparesis a problem for people with diabetes is that it can greatly hinder your efforts at blood glucose control. If you can't predict how quickly your food will be digested, your insulin or medication could work too quickly or too slowly.

Symptoms of gastroparesis may include:

· Nausea
· Vomiting
· Abdominal bloating
· Weight loss
· Premature feeling of fullness.

Dealing with Gastroparesis

People with gastroparesis who take insulin frequently need to adjust their dosage. Insulin lispro (Humalog) may be recommended, since it starts working within minutes and peaks within an hour or two. If you have gastroparesis, your doctor can provide specific recommendations for insulin therapy for your particular situation.

Adjustments to diet are also usually necessary to ease gastroparesis. High-fat and high-fibre foods are discouraged, since they slow digestion. Your doctor may recommend smaller, more frequent meals, or replacing some meals with liquid-based nutrition. In cases where vomiting is so extreme that you are having trouble keeping food down altogether, parenteral or jejunostomy (tube) feeding may be required.

Jejunostomy involves insertion of a feeding tube through the abdomen and into the small intestine. A liquid nutritional compound is then administered through the tube. Parenteral nutrition uses an intravenous line directly into the bloodstream to provide vital nutrients. It is usually used only as a temporary measure while treatment by other means is stabilized.

For cases that are unresponsive to dietary changes, injections of botulinum toxin (botox) into the sphincter of the pylorus (the opening connecting the stomach to the small intestine) may be attempted in an effort to relax the opening to let food pass through more readily.

Up to 50 per cent of people with diabetes develop gastroparesis, although the vast majority will experience it only to a mild extent. It occurs most frequently in people with Type 1 diabetes, although it does also occur in people with Type 2.

Medication may also be prescribed to try to speed up digestion. Commonly prescribed gastroparesis medications include metaclopramide (Maxalon), domperidone (Motilium) and erythromycin (an antibiotic that can speed stomach emptying).

Enterra Therapy (Medtronic) is a device that uses electrical impulses to stimulate digestion by the stomach. It has been described as a pacemaker for the stomach and has been successful in treating chronic gastroparesis in some patients for whom drug therapy was not effective.

Skin Problems

There are a number of different skin conditions that can affect people with diabetes. Nerve and small blood vessel damage can make dry skin worse. Keeping the skin well hydrated is important because any cracks or fissures could easily become infected. In addition to being uncomfortable, the itchiness of dry skin may cause a scratch or abrasion that also poses an infection risk.

Use a humidifier in the home and office, and avoid exposure to harsh detergents and household cleaners that are notorious for drying out skin. If you keep a bottle of hand lotion next to the soap at the kitchen and bathroom sinks, you'll be more likely to remember to use it after each hand-washing. Make sure the soap you use for washing is mild.

Tougher areas of the skin, such as the soles of the feet, may benefit from a moisturizing lotion containing urea (for moisture) and alpha-hydroxy, or AHA (for sloughing off dead skin). It's a good idea to check any new products with your doctor or diabetes specialist nurse first. Using baby powder in the armpits, between the toes and on other moisture-prone skin fold areas can help to prevent fungal infections.

People with diabetes frequently develop thickened, shiny areas of skin that are caused by changes to the collagen fibres. A tendency towards yellow-tinted skin and nails, too, may be triggered by collagen changes (although the cause of this phenomenon isn't completely understood).

Other skin conditions that are common in people with diabetes include the following:

- **Acanthosis nigricans:** Dark, thickened brown patches in the folds of the skin that are common in overweight people with insulin resistance and Type 2 diabetes.
- **Bacterial infections:** Staphyloccus or streptococcus infections in the skin that may appear as styes, boils or cellulitis.
- **Fungal infections:** These usually occur in warm, moist areas such as skin folds. Candidiasis (yeast infection), tinea pedis (athlete's foot or ringworm) and tinea cruris (jock itch or ringworm) are all common fungal infections.
- **Diabetic dermopathy:** Brown, scaly, rounded patches on the skin that frequently appear on the shins and usually heal on their own.
- **Necrobiosis lipoidica diabeticorum:** Changes in the collagen of the skin that cause large, raised, red, shiny and sometimes itchy spots. If the spots rupture, they will require proper wound care.

Several other, less common, conditions that may occur in the presence of uncontrolled high blood glucose levels include bullosis diabeticorum (diabetic blisters) and eruptive xanthomatosis (small, yellow, red-ringed bumps), most commonly due to high lipids. Both of these conditions usually resolve themselves once blood glucose levels are brought back under control.

Chapter 16

The Diabetic Foot

What have your feet got to do with diabetes, you ask? A lot. In time, high blood glucose levels can deaden your nerves and clog up the cardiovascular system, making neuropathy and peripheral vascular disease a real danger to the feet. And as someone with diabetes, your body is slower to heal and prone to infection, so small blisters and abrasions can turn into serious complications if not treated promptly and properly.

Treat Your Feet Right

It has been estimated that the average person walks about 184,500km (115,000 miles) in a lifetime (over four times around the Equator, if you're counting). With all that walking, your feet get put through a lot of wear and tear. For most people, the pain of a blister or cut is a signal to get off your feet and let them heal. But if you have diabetic neuropathy (nerve damage) in your feet, the pain signal is impaired or gone altogether, and you may not notice an injury until you actually see it.

My 12-year-old daughter has Type 1 diabetes. Do we really have to worry about her feet at such a young age?

While children and teenagers with Type 1 diabetes are less likely to develop foot problems than adults, proper foot care is a good habit to get into early. As they grow older, nerve and circulatory impairment will become a bigger risk. In general, people with Type 2 diabetes are at greater risk of foot complications simply because they often have extended periods of uncontrolled hyperglycaemia before diagnosis.

Daily Foot Check

It only takes a minute to check your feet for signs of abrasions, blisters or other problems, and it could save you serious medical problems down the line. Make it a part of your daily routine, either as you get dressed for the day, at shower time or as you get ready for bed. Before you know it, it will become a healthy habit.

You should give your entire foot the once-over, and check between your toes. If you have flexibility and/or vision problems and have trouble seeing everything adequately, ask a family member for help. A flexible, magnified mirror can help you see those hard-to-reach spots.

Blisters, Corns and Calluses

Do not burst or break blisters, as this will increase your risk of infection. Keep a close eye on the wounds. If they start to get worse, exhibit signs of infection (such as pus, redness and warmth or odour), or don't look as if they are healing within a day or so, call your doctor immediately for further instruction.

Keep your feet moisturized to avoid cracks caused by dryness. Try not to apply lotion between the toes, as it can breed fungal growth or infection. Peripheral neuropathy can cause a 10 per cent decrease in skin moisture in the feet, so if you have any degree of PN, take extra care to use skin cream regularly.

If you develop corns or calluses, you're better off letting a podiatrist treat them. If you have PN, do *not* try to remove corns or calluses with cutting implements or chemical treatments on your own. You should have access to a hospital-based podiatrist if there is no community podiatrist available in your area. Sometimes, designated members of the primary care team (at your GP's surgery) are trained in giving specialist footcare advice to people with diabetes, but ask your doctor for a referral to a podiatrist if necessary – particularly if you are need of treatment. A pumice stone may be used only with your doctor's approval.

Clipping Correctly

To prevent ingrown toenails, clip your nails straight across. Don't cut too close to the skin line, to avoid an accidental slice into your skin. You can smooth out any sharp corners with an emery board. Thick or discoloured toenails should be checked out by your doctor or podiatrist, as they could be a sign of a fungal infection.

The Right Equipment

Keeping your feet in good condition means making sure you have proper protection against the elements. The only time you should be going barefoot is in bed and in the shower. Make sure your shoes and socks or stockings are appropriate for your needs. An extra investment may be required, but in the long run the comfort and reduced risk of complications will be well worth the added expense.

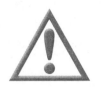

Invest in a pair of aqua shoes if you visit the beach. The sand can be full of hidden hazards such as broken glass and sharp seashells, and on a hot day the possibility of burning your feet is a real danger. Never go without foot protection in the water, either.

Shoes Off the Rack

You have several options for shoes, ranging from regular, off-the-rack footwear to custom-made prescription shoes. If you don't have any diagnosed podiatric conditions, you can probably fulfil your footwear needs at a standard shoe shop. However, there are some sensible shoe tips you should follow to keep your feet safe:

·   **Stay grounded.** High heels are not good for your feet and can cause blisters.
·   **On your toes.** Open-toed shoes also present a hazard, as they leave a good portion of your foot exposed. Leave the sandals and stay safe.
·   **Get fit.** If at all possible, have a trained salesperson check the fit of your shoes in the store.
·   **Wiggle room.** Properly fitting shoes should leave room for your toes to move freely, and be wide and long enough for a firm yet comfortable fit.
·   **Breathing room.** Leather or canvas uppers are your best bet for shoes that allow your feet to breathe, not sweat.

Shoes by Prescription

If you have existing foot problems, you'll probably need something a little more customized. Depth shoes are special therapeutic footwear that have extra room for the toes and for any orthotic inserts. If you have foot problems such as hammertoes or bunions, depth shoes may be appropriate for you.

Orthotics are prescription devices that are inserted into shoes to relieve pressure and provide extra cushion and support. To produce a custom fit, your podiatrist may take special casts of your feet. Some newer orthotics production technology uses a sensor mat that you walk on to provide a computer-generated view of what portions of your feet bear the greatest load. Special software then designs the specifications for orthotics that are made to order. Your podiatrist or a specialist called an orthotist or pedorthist (a person trained in the design, fabrication and fit of orthotic inserts) can help fit you for orthotics.

Custom-moulded shoes may be required for some people with diabetes-related foot deformities such as cases of Charcot foot. Again, these customized shoes are obtained through a podiatrist or orthotist, who performs a special casting to fit the shoes properly.

Comfort should be a prerequisite for any new pair of shoes you purchase. However, it's still a good idea to break them in gradually to avoid blisters. Wear them around the house for a short period daily for about a week until they start to feel 'lived in'.

Sock Sense

Even the best-fitting shoes won't do much good if you're wearing threadbare or hole-riddled socks. Lay a good foundation with thick, well-cushioned socks that are seamless (to prevent any friction blisters) and wick moisture away from the foot. Cotton, cotton-polyester or acrylic blends are all good choices.

There are also some newer treated fabrics and blends out on the market, such as Teflon and antimicrobial fibres, designed to prevent blisters and infection. Since socks are a relatively small investment, it's a good idea to try out a variety until you find a type that suits you for style and comfort.

Tight and restrictive elastic bands (garters, for example) can cut off circulation, but some degree of compression built into the sock construction can be supportive and help to protect against deep-vein thrombosis. Other people, particularly those with oedema (swollen feet), may do better with a loose-fitting sock. Your podiatrist can advise you on what's right for your particular needs.

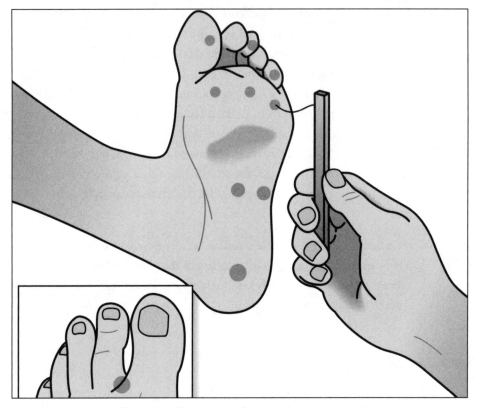

▲ The monofilament test for peripheral neuropathy.

Monofilament Test

Peripheral neuropathy (PN), or nerve damage of the extremities, is one of the most common complications of diabetes (at least 50 per cent of all people with the disease develop it at some point). Symptoms include burning, tingling, numbness, a prickly sensation (such as pins and needles), and muscle weakness. Neuropathy is the result of chronically high blood sugars, so the best way to prevent it is to maintain good glucose control.

To check for neuropathy, your doctor should perform a monofilament test – a measure of the sensation in your feet – at least once a year, as part of your Annual Review. In this simple yet sensitive evaluation, the monofilament, which is a piece of plastic fibre that resembles fishing line, is touched against various parts of the sole of your foot, and your ability to feel it at varying pressure is assessed. It is sometimes called the 10g monofilament test because the fibre is calibrated to bend to 10g of pressure. Your doctor may also use a tuning fork on the bottoms of your feet to see if you can sense the vibration.

Nerve-conduction studies or velocity tests, which use electrodes to stimulate nerves and then measure the resulting impulses, are a less frequently used, more sophisticated method of diagnosing some neuropathies. Electromyography (EMG), which uses thin needles inserted into the muscles to measure electrical impulses, may also be prescribed. These latter two tests can be painful, and may not be ordered unless there is some question about the diagnosis.

Avoid the use of hot-water bottles, heating pads and other foot-warming devices if you have neuropathy. You could inadvertently burn yourself, so stick with a warm pair of socks. And never go without at least a pair of slippers on, even for a late-night trek to the toilet, as you run the risk of stabbing your foot or tripping and injuring your exposed foot.

When to See a Podiatrist

Your doctor should refer you to a podiatrist – who has specialist training in the physiology and medical care of the foot and ankle – if you show any signs of developing problems with your feet. Both the blood supply and the nerve supply to the feet will be regularly assessed, and any skin changes carefully monitored.

If you have had diagnosed structural, nerve or skin problems with your feet, a podiatrist should be on your diabetes care team, and you should see him at least every three months. Foot ulcers, in particular, require specialized wound care to avoid infection and, in the ultimate case, possible amputation.

In addition to the regular tests for neuropathy described previously, your podiatrist may assess the pulse and blood pressure of the foot and ankle and the temperature of your feet to screen for circulatory problems. Ultrasound or Doppler may be used to check blood flow.

Add diabetic foot problems to the long list of negative health effects of smoking. Smoking tobacco constricts your blood vessels, which can make circulatory problems worse and restrict blood flow to your feet.

Charcot Foot or Joint

Charcot foot or joint, also called neuropathic arthropathy, is a podiatric condition that occurs in an estimated 9–30 per cent of people suffering from diabetic peripheral neuropathy. It is caused by a breakdown of the joints and bones that goes unnoticed because of nerve damage and results in deformities of the bones of the feet. The condition is usually treated by a podiatrist or an orthopaedist.

Typical signs of Charcot foot include extreme swelling, warmth of the skin and redness. Because these are also signs of infection, cellulitis or deep-vein thrombosis, an X-ray examination is needed to confirm the diagnosis.

The Healing Process

In order to heal properly, a Charcot foot is usually immobilized in a contact cast, which is replaced periodically in order to inspect the foot. This foot-to-upper-leg cast cushions and protects the foot, and in many cases you may be able to walk on it with the help of crutches or a cane. However, some patients may be instructed to stay off their feet completely while the cast is on.

The cast may need to stay on as long as six months while the foot heals; after it is removed, a leg brace may be required. Frequently, pressure ulcers form as a result of the foot deformity and consequent redistribution of weight. Reconstructive surgery may be required in extreme cases where ulcers become a recurring problem. Physiotherapy can also help you regain motion and learn adaptive exercise techniques.

Diabetes is the leading cause of lower-extremity amputation in the UK, but at least half of all amputations could be prevented with early intervention and proper foot and skin care.

Diabetic Foot Ulcers

If you've ever had local anaesthetic at the dentist, you know how it feels to try to talk or eat afterwards – rather like knitting with boxing gloves on. People who have lost the sensation in their feet have a similar experience. Neuropathy often causes an unnatural and awkward stride, which puts repeated pressure on the same spot of your foot. Over time, this area will callus and may eventually develop into a pressure ulcer. Other diabetic foot ulcers may be caused by poor circulation in your legs and feet. Beyond practising good foot care, the best thing you can do to prevent limb-threatening complications from ulcers is detect them early and treat them properly.

How They Happen

Most ulcers form on the bottom of the foot, although shoes that don't fit well can cause sores and subsequent ulcers on the top of the foot or the ankle. Usually ulcers start as a callus, small sore, abrasion or blister that would be no big deal for someone without diabetes. However, high blood glucose levels, poor circulation and nerve damage are a recipe for ulceration in people with diabetes.

There are two categories of foot ulcers: vascular and neuropathic (or pressure) ulcers. The former is caused by peripheral vascular disease; the latter is the result of the loss of sensation that accompanies peripheral neuropathy. People who have PN may put increased pressure on the same area of their foot repeatedly, resulting in callusing at first, and eventually in ulceration. Ulcers caused by PVD are usually painful, while those caused by PN are not.

Keep those feet moving to ward off vascular ulcers and promote good circulation. Exercise (low-impact if you have foot problems), avoid sitting with your legs crossed for more than a few minutes at a time, and periodically stretch your legs and toes. Putting up your feet when you're at rest can also help blood flow.

Treatment

Infection is the primary risk with foot ulcers, so proper wound care is essential. Ulcers should remain moist and covered in a breathable dressing at all times (except when changing bandages). Oxygen is essential to the healing process. An antibiotic ointment may be applied if infection is present. Oral antibiotic medication should also be prescribed. If you have a pressure ulcer, debridement – removal of callused, dead skin – may also be performed by the podiatrist.

Your doctor may also prescribe one of several new 'human-based' ulcer treatments, such as Regranex (Janssen-Cilag). Regranex is a gel containing platelet growth factors that promote healing and new skin growth.

Ulcers that are the result of PVD may show up on the lower leg as well as the foot. The toes are also a common location, and if circulation is poor enough, tissue necrosis (tissue death) or gangrene may be evident in the surrounding blackened skin. These patients may need an arterial bypass to restore blood flow to their feet and legs.

Osteomyelitis, or bone infection, may occur if infection in the ulcer spreads deeply enough. This is usually diagnosed with a bone scan or magnetic resonance imaging (MRI), and is treated with intravenous antibiotic therapy.

Chapter 17

Kids and Diabetes

Growing up with diabetes is a challenge for both child and parent. Dealing with doctors, blood tests and injections, school issues, medical supplies and everything else that comes with the diabetes package is a full-time job in itself. But as your child grows, you'll find her able to take more responsibility for her own care.

The Littlest Patients: Infants and Toddlers

As any parent can attest, not knowing how to help your hurting child is a horrible feeling. When your very young child has diabetes, she can't tell you if she's 'feeling low' or needs to check her blood glucose. But just as parents develop a sense of a 'hungry cry', as opposed to a 'wet cry', you will become attuned to the signs your child gives about how she's feeling.

A paediatric diabetologist is a doctor who has specialized in treating diabetes in children. It is likely that your GP will refer you to see one of these specialists, who are usually based at a hospital. You may also see a paediatric diabetes specialist nurse, who has also specialized in treating diabetes in children. You can rest assured that your child's health care team will know all about the particular problems faced by children with diabetes – and the problems faced by their parents, too.

Recognizing Signs and Symptoms

The same symptoms that occur in older kids and adults signalling the possibility of Type 1 diabetes apply to infants and toddlers; the difference is that since their verbal communication skills are limited, you probably won't recognize them as quickly. In addition, symptoms such as fatigue are hard to discern in a baby who sleeps a good deal of the day anyway. The positive news is that most parents, particularly new ones, will take a 'rather safe than sorry' attitude and take an inconsolable infant or toddler to the doctor to work out what's wrong quickly, rather than waiting around for things to worsen. If your child is at risk of Type 1 diabetes, look for the following symptoms:

· Excessive wet nappies
· Nappy rash that doesn't go away quickly or keeps recurring
· Constant hunger and/or thirst
· Irritability or fussiness that doesn't seem related to colic
· Sleeping more than usual.

Detecting Highs and Lows

Recognizing high and low blood glucose levels may be hard when a diabetes diagnosis is new in your very young child. Fortunately, you have the best tool for making sure things are in balance right at your fingertips – a glucose meter. If your child is acting the least bit out of sorts, always check glucose levels first. It may not be her diabetes, but if it is, you want to find out quickly and treat it fast. Talk to your child's doctor about an appropriate amount of carbohydrates to treat her hypos. As a general rule, kids under the age of six require 5–10g of a fast-acting carbohydrate if their blood glucose is low.

If you have an infant or toddler with diabetes, have an oral syringe on hand to administer a fast-acting liquid carbohydrate such as syrup if a hypo occurs and your baby refuses a bottle of juice. Glucose gel in a tube (Hypostop) can also work for more cooperative eaters. Never feed a child who has lost consciousness because of the risk of choking or aspiration, and never give an infant a glucose tablet or a hard sweet.

Glucose Monitoring

Glucose checks are a tough job for parents, especially for very young children who don't have the capacity to understand why they must be poked and prodded. You can make it a little easier by buying an alternate site meter, which allows you to test on less sensitive areas, such as the forearm. You may also be able to prick the heel instead of the fingers. Talk to your child's doctor for her or his specific recommendations, and try out different meters until you find one that works well for you. Both you and your child will eventually get used to testing.

On Eating and Insulin

Small children have notoriously unpredictable appetites. They can go for days eating very little, and then suddenly down a whole plateful of macaroni cheese in the blink of an eye. Of course, if you don't know what your child is going to wolf down or push away at the next meal, it makes giving insulin a bit difficult. For this reason, your doctor may recommend rapid-acting insulin to be administered immediately following a meal, to correctly cover the carbohydrates and avoid highs or lows.

Insulin injections can be traumatic for young children, but there are several injection aids available to make the job easier on both of you. Your doctor can prescribe a topical anaesthetic cream to numb the injection site, and a device called an Inject-Ease can be used with a standard syringe to both hide the needle and minimize pain by facilitating a rapid injection.

Taking Diabetes to School

Sending your child off to school for the first time is particularly tough for parents. In addition to all the usual parental worries, you have your child's diabetes to think about. The good news is that many, many others have gone before you and have blazed the trail, so to speak, for your child's rights in the classroom.

Diabetes UK can provide general information for school staff; it will be up to you to work out the specifics, which might require some negotiation on your part. A record card (template available from Diabetes UK) with vital medical information (see below) and a passport-sized photo may be of assistance to the school. If you face uncooperative school staff, there are specific legal protections in place to ensure that your child gets appropriate medical care and fair, non-discriminatory treatment while in the classroom.

For the Record

Vital information that the school may require includes:

- **Blood glucose monitoring requirements.** Spell out how often checks should occur, under what circumstances extra checks might be required (i.e. exercise), logging procedures and how the meter and supplies should be stored.
- **Insulin requirements.** List insulin doses, when they should be taken,

how much insulin is required for specific glucose values or for covering a meal, and how to properly store insulin. If your child uses an insulin pump, include information on that as well.

· **Meals, snacks and fluids.** A dietary plan for meals eaten at school should describe your child's recommended carbohydrate intake for lunch and snacks, when he or she should eat, and also how to handle special occasions (i.e. birthday cakes at school).

· **Recognizing and treating highs and lows.** The plan should explain the signs of both hypoglycaemia (low blood glucose) and hyperglycaemia (high blood glucose), and how to promptly and correctly treat both. Explicit directions on the administration of a glucagon shot should also be included, and staff should be trained in its use as well.

· **Ketone testing.** Explain when ketone testing is appropriate and how the procedure works.

· **Contact information.** This probably goes without saying, but make sure your record includes your full contact information, a back-up emergency contact, and a back-up for your back-up. Someone should be reachable at all times.

Dealing With Discrimination

Every child will probably have to deal with some form of discrimination in his or her life, usually due to an ignorance of what Type 1 diabetes is all about. It can be as simple as denying a child a biscuit in the cafeteria, or as overt as denying self-monitoring for a child who is perfectly capable of performing it.

Although most children with diabetes would not consider themselves to be disabled, the Disability Discrimination Act 1995 (DDA) does offer children with diabetes legal protection from discrimination.

Local Education Authorities (LEAs), schools (public and private) and higher education facilities are all legally obliged to ensure that pupils with diabetes are not treated less favourably, and that 'reasonable' adjustments are made to ensure that they are not put at a disadvantage.

If you feel that discrimination has occurred or is occurring, then you will need to figure out how best to resolve the problem. You may wish to pursue the matter through formal DDA procedures, or you might prefer to take a more informal approach first. Since discrimination often arises out of ignorance, it may be that all that is needed is some education and enlightenment. However, if you need assistance in any way, call the Disability Rights Commission Helpline (see Appendix A).

Educating the Educators

If your child's school is not up to date with the needs of children with diabetes, then some training may be in order, and it's in your best interest to get involved in the process early on. Ask to attend any teaching sessions the school sets up, to ensure their accuracy and provide practical input on how the information specifically applies to your child.

If your child's school has a nurse on duty who will help your child with his diabetes care, schedule a meeting with her to go over your child's particular treatment needs and to ensure that she knows exactly what to do in case of a hypoglycaemic emergency. The nurse should also attend any diabetes training sessions.

Your child's school may ask you for input or assistance in coordinating teacher training. This is a good opportunity to get your child's diabetes specialist nurse in to meet all the teaching staff and support personnel (i.e. bus driver, cafeteria assistants, playground personnel) that your child will have contact with, in order to make them aware of her medical needs and to provide them with an accurate, working knowledge of what Type 1 diabetes is really all about.

School personnel who have contact with your child should be trained in all aspects of diabetes care. Even the most competent child may have situations where his blood glucose drops too low and he needs assistance with a check and/or a quick fix of glucose.

Treatment in the Classroom

Your child's school is not legally obligated to allow blood glucose testing in the classroom, and your son or daughter may be required to go to the nurse's office or another place to check glucose levels. However, for older children who are both capable of carrying out a check themselves and comfortable with doing it in class, it is usually in the best interest of all involved if the child is allowed to do checks right there in the classroom. Your child will miss less class time – if they are feeling low they don't have to use up precious time travelling to the nurse's office – and it is less disruptive to the entire class if he or she can discreetly check without leaving the room.

There should always be a fast-acting glucose snack available in your child's classroom for her immediate use. You will have primary responsibility for keeping an adequate supply available for her, as well as keeping unexpired meter strips and supplies, insulin and everything else she needs in stock.

School Sports

Sports are another area where children may be treated differently because they have diabetes. Kids who want to get involved with team or individual sports should not be dissuaded or automatically excluded on the basis of their diabetes alone. With appropriate precautions, your child can excel in just about anything she wishes.

If your child is participating in school sports, her coach should be involved in diabetes training, along with her other teachers. It's particularly important that coaches realize the signs of hypoglycaemia, since exercise may induce a hypo, and know how to treat it appropriately.

Coaches or instructors of team or individual sports that take place outside of the school setting also need proper education about your child's medical needs. If you can, consider volunteering to coach or help out with the team to make the learning curve a little easier.

Coming of Age With Diabetes

The preteenage and teenage years are a rocky time for all kids; as their social identities emerge, they start such eternally awkward rituals as going on dates, and they pull away from their parents to find their own sense of self and establish their independence. This is a particularly tricky time for adolescents with diabetes, who may be desperately trying to find a way to fit in when their blood glucose checks, insulin injections and eating habits all say 'I'm different'.

The hormonal changes of puberty also take a toll on diabetes control in and of themselves, increasing overall insulin resistance. Girls and boys face a sea change in their bodies that makes control a bit more elusive than normal. Things will stabilize after a time. (For more on dealing with puberty, see Chapters 18 and 19.)

This is also an age for experimentation with drugs, alcohol and smoking, all things that will affect your child's blood glucose control in ways he or she is not accustomed to. Worse, drugs and alcohol can have an impact on your child's perception of low blood glucose levels and impair his ability to make good decisions.

Now is the time to have a frank talk about drugs, alcohol and cigarettes. Your child needs to know how it will affect his diabetes, and what precautions he needs to take if he does try any of these things. Giving him this information is not the same as saying you approve of his experimentation with drugs or alcohol; in fact, he also needs to know explicitly that you don't want him using them at all. But since adolescence is often filled with bad decisions as teenagers try to find their own identity, educating your child while accepting the possibility could literally save his life.

Sex is another area where a candid discussion is necessary. Your adolescent needs to know about birth control and the risks of unprotected sex in terms of sexually transmitted diseases and unwanted pregnancy. Again, you don't have to condone it, but you do need to provide vital information.

A full explanation of the risks both mother and child face during pregnancy when blood glucose levels are not well controlled is in order. Keep it balanced. Make sure that your teenager recognizes that when she is older and ready to start a family, a safe and healthy *planned* pregnancy is achievable.

Handling Special Days

Birthdays, special treats, sleepovers – sometimes it seems like childhood is one big food festival. It's hard to deny your child special treats when all her peers are digging in. Fortunately, with insulin adjustments and good planning, your child can partake in some of the sweet treats of childhood in moderation.

Birthday Parties

When a birthday invitation arrives, talk to the host parents in good time to find out what's on the menu. If it's something your child is particularly sensitive to, bring a special snack. Make sure the parent knows what amount of cake and/or ice-cream is allowed. You may have to accompany your child to most parties, even when he surpasses the age where most parents hang around. With a full list of other guests to attend to, you can't reasonably expect the party hosts to attend to your child's medical needs, especially if the birthday child is a classroom acquaintance and the parents are largely unfamiliar with diabetes and your child's special needs.

If attending the party becomes an issue with your child and her growing sense of independence, assure her that you'll fade into the background as much as possible, except when your help is needed. When the celebration takes place at a public venue such as an ice-skating rink or a cinema, this is a bit easier on both of you.

Think about bringing siblings and making a separate family affair out of it so you're almost not even there. This usually works out best for all involved – you aren't hanging around, making your child feel self-conscious, it gives the host parents peace of mind to know you are in the area should your help be needed, and you feel better knowing your child is nearby. Your other kids and/or your partner also get a day of fun out of it, so everyone wins.

Overnight Trips

The first solo sleepover can be nerve-wracking for both you and the host parents. Kids old enough for sleepovers and overnight trips are typically at least starting to manage some of their own diabetes care, which helps. Spend some time with the parents before the event to give them a briefing on what your child might potentially need, and make yourself available via the phone for any questions they might have during the visit. Provide them with a one-page sheet with all treatment basics; trouble signs will be helpful as well.

Finding Babysitters

Caring for a child with chronic illness takes a big emotional and physical toll on parents, and you, too, need an occasional break from it all. It's true that caregivers, especially for small children with diabetes, can be difficult to find. Some adults feel overwhelmed by the responsibility of caring for a child (think about how you felt when your child was first diagnosed). Others worry about the legal liability should something go wrong under their care. Fear is a big factor in many people's unwillingness to babysit children with diabetes, and this is often the easiest obstacle to overcome.

Don't give up on finding a babysitter out of hand because you've been unsuccessful before. And don't stay with your child constantly because you live in fear of the worst possible scenario happening when you're away.

If you have relatives nearby, they are a natural choice for baby-sitting duties. If not, check friends and neighbours for potential candidates. You need someone responsible, caring and cool-headed – the same qualities you would look for in a babysitter if your child didn't have diabetes. When you make the first contact, explain up front that your child does have diabetes and has some special needs. Then invite your potential babysitter over for an afternoon (or even several afternoons) to interact and watch your child with you around as back-up, to see what caring for your child really entails. Often the babysitter will find that the reality is not even close to what his imagination had cooked up.

When you leave your child with a babysitter, always pass on a list of emergency contact numbers (including your child's doctor's surgery), along with detailed instructions on your child's diabetes care. If you have an extra copy of your child's school record card around, photocopying it for babysitters is a good idea since it should contain all essential treatment information.

Kids Being Kids

Children with diabetes who live in rural areas often are the only child in their school, or possibly even their community, who has to deal with the special issues related to living with this disease. Even children in more populated areas can sometimes feel alone and isolated, as can their parents.

What About Diabetes Camp?

Diabetes camp can be a great adventure for children – teaching them management skills that will last a lifetime and, equally as important, giving them the chance to spend a few weeks with peers who share their concerns and experiences.

Diabetes UK run a series of summer camps for children across the UK. They also run a number of Outward Bound courses for teenagers and young adults, which prove very popular. Most are, of course, summer programmes, and many of the helpers at these camps also have diabetes and can relate to your children as a mentor and a diabetes peer and/or role model. In addition to all the typical summer camp activities, such as swimming, canoeing and craftmaking, your child will learn more about her or his diabetes and how to care for it.

Finally, you can have a care-giving respite with the peace of mind that your child is somewhere where you know his or her diabetes will be well taken care of.

Type 2 and Kids – a Growing Problem

A 2002 study on obesity and children in the *New England Journal of Medicine*, published in the USA, brought to light the growing problem of kids, weight and insulin resistance, finding a strong association between childhood obesity and impaired glucose tolerance.

The latest data from the Health Survey for England (2002) showed 18 per cent of schoolchildren to be overweight and a further 6 per cent to be obese. Extrapolating from these figures, researchers have estimated that 1,400 children in the UK could have Type 2 diabetes, and over 20,000 children could have impaired glucose tolerance (IGT). Many overweight or obese children may already have Type 2 diabetes, but don't know it yet.

Apart from Type 2 diabetes, childhood obesity can lead to adult medical issues, such as atherosclerosis, hypertension, respiratory infections and sleep apnea.

Studies show that sugary, sweet soft drinks can increase the likelihood of a child becoming obese by up to 60 per cent. The extra calories in sweet drinks such as colas and fizzy drinks can cause significant weight gain if not consumed in moderation, so look at sugar-free or diet soda alternatives.

Weight Control and Exercise

If your child is at risk of developing Type 2 diabetes and has issues with weight, diet and exercise should be your immediate defence plan. In this situation, your doctor may refer you to a state registered dietician who can formulate a medically sound weight-loss programme that is tailored to your child's specific needs. A dietician can also be of great help when it comes to creating a balanced meal plan for your child.

Every child, no matter what her level of athleticism, should be encouraged to get out and get moving. If she's interested, get her involved in some team sports and/or outdoor activities. If she isn't into athletics, activities such as bicycle and scooter riding, rollerblading, walking, swimming or dancing are good, non-competitive ways to get fit. The important thing is to find something that interests her so that it becomes something she looks forward to instead of dreading.

Keep food itself in perspective and treat it as fuel, not entertainment, comfort, love or reward. Using treats to make a child feel better instead of communicating about her problems turns food into an inappropriate substitute for affection, and can sabotage self-esteem and self-sufficiency.

Diabetes is a family disease, whether it be Type 1 or Type 2. Kids can't be expected to diet and exercise if their parents and siblings are living a fast-food, couch-potato lifestyle. Plan meals and group activities that everyone can enjoy together.

If your child has been diagnosed with Type 2 diabetes, now is the time to get him on the path to healthy food attitudes and fitness to get both bad habits and his diabetes under control. What your child learns now will serve him well for the rest of his life.

Chapter 18

Special Issues for Women

Feeling as if you're in a permanent state of PMS – even if you're well past menopause? The hormonal tides of puberty, pregnancy, menstruation and menopause are each yet another seismic force to contend with as you try to maintain balance and control of your diabetes. Remember that treatment is not a static thing – 'adapt, adapt, adapt' will be your motto as you move through the stages of diabetes care.

At Puberty

The barrage of hormones, social turmoil, fashion crises and other adolescent dramas that spells puberty can also spell trouble for your teenager's (or preteenager's) diabetes control. Issues of poor self-image and of wanting to fit in with peers by acting and eating as they do may raise glucose levels, either through non-compliance with treatment or as a stress response. Hormonal changes, which magnify all of the preceding and can increase the need for insulin, compound the problem.

I've heard skipping my insulin is an easy way to lose some weight. Can I do it if I don't eat much?

Skipping your insulin can be deadly. While you might lose a little, DKA is a very real risk, along with all the other hazards of poor control. Your body probably needs more insulin now because of the hormonal changes of puberty. It's really important to talk to someone about how you're feeling. Start with your doctor – a good one won't judge you or make you feel bad – she'll try to help.

Girls going through puberty will have an increased need for insulin as oestrogen and progesterone production rev up with menarche (the first menstrual period). The peak age for Type 1 diabetes diagnosis for girls is between the ages of 10 and 12, when puberty is often in full bloom.

At Risk of Eating Disorders

Eating disorders are more than twice as common in teenage girls with diabetes than those without. Girls with eating disorders may skip their insulin dosage – a practice called insulin omission – in an effort to lose weight. By doing so, they are also at a higher risk for developing diabetic ketoacidosis (DKA) and poor overall control (as measured by HbA1c levels).

Diabetes and Menstruation

If you are a premenopausal woman with diabetes, you may notice a rise in blood glucose levels as your menstrual period draws closer. The rise in oestrogen and progesterone levels that occurs towards the end of the cycle (about a week before menstruation) can increase insulin resistance, causing a rise in glucose levels. In other women with diabetes, this hormonal change may actually increase insulin sensitivity, triggering lower blood glucose levels. And in the true 'one-size-fits-none' nature of diabetes, some women may experience no changes at all.

Monitoring your glucose levels throughout your monthly cycle can help you understand whether hormones are having an impact on your diabetes control (yet one more thing to keep in your blood glucose log). Discuss your results with your doctor or diabetes specialist nurse. Adjustments in medication, insulin, exercise and diet may be necessary to bring your glucose levels back to normal during this time.

Pregnancy: Treatment for Two

Having a baby is not a decision to be entered into lightly for anyone. For women with diabetes, the decision may be even more difficult because of the demands placed on their body, the necessity for painstaking control before and during the pregnancy, and the potential for developing or worsening diabetic complications in the whole pregnancy and birth process.

Some complications of diabetes, including retinopathy, nephropathy and neuropathy, can get worse in pregnancy. Your doctor will talk to you about your specific risks as part of preconception planning. Tests that may be ordered during preconception planning include:

· Thyroid (TSH; for Type 1)
· Kidney function
· Comprehensive eye examination
· Cardiovascular screening.

Diabetic retinopathy is one condition that pregnancy may make worse. Diabetes UK Care Recommendations say that in addition to a dilated eye examination during preconception planning, women who become pregnant should have a comprehensive eye test in the first trimester and close follow-up throughout pregnancy if retinopathy is present.

Control Before Conception

When it comes to having a successful pregnancy with Type 1 or Type 2 diabetes, planning is everything. Achieving good blood glucose control before conception is the best way to ensure a good outcome for both you and your child. Diabetes UK recommends that women who plan on becoming pregnant strive for an HbA1c level of less than 7 per cent, and pre- and postprandial glucose readings as outlined in the following table.

Recommended Glucose Readings for Women Planning to Conceive	
Test	**Range**
Before meals Capillary whole blood glucose	<5.6 mmol/l
Before meals Capillary plasma glucose	4.4–6.1 mmol/l
2 hours after meals Capillary whole blood glucose	<7.8 mmol/l
2 hours after meals Capillary plasma glucose	<8.6 mmol/l

If you take drugs for hypertension or other diabetic complications, your doctor will discuss your options with you, as many are not recommended for pregnancy. Drug therapy that is contraindicated in pregnancy includes oral diabetes medications, and these will have to be stopped and replaced with insulin therapy (which is considered safe in pregnancy). Starting insulin before you try to conceive will help you become accustomed to the routine and make appropriate dosage adjustments for optimal control.

Ideally, blood glucose will be stabilized at the target goal, or as close as possible to it, for several months before you try to conceive. Adjustments to insulin and other aspects of your treatment will have to be made during pregnancy, too, which is why it's important to continue to stay in close contact with both your diabetes care team (who may be hospital-based) and antenatal care team (who may be hospital-based, or may be your GP and local midwife).

Staying Healthy During Pregnancy

Once you become pregnant, your GP may refer you to an antenatal clinic that specializes in high-risk pregnancies. Your antenatal care and diabetes care should be closely coordinated, with all of the health care professionals communicating with each other and, of course, with you.

Your insulin needs will go up in pregnancy, as your placenta starts to manufacture hormones that increase your insulin resistance. Frequent glucose checks during this time are critical, and your diabetes doctor and specialist nurse will help you to adjust your daily insulin doses to keep on top of things. Your doctor will also request frequent HbA1c testing (once a month at the very least).

Your Baby and Diabetes

If you are able to keep your blood glucose well controlled during pregnancy, your baby's risk of complications is reduced dramatically. Tight control in the first trimester in particular is important, because this is the critical time when the organ systems are developing in the foetus.

Babies born to mothers with diabetes have a greater chance of being born large for birth weight. This is because the foetus converts extra glucose into body fat in the womb. The condition, called macrosomia, puts newborns at risk for unplanned Caesarian section birth and shoulder dystocia (getting wedged in the birth canal during delivery).

During labour you will most probably have an insulin and glucose drip so that your blood glucose levels can be kept closely in check. This works on a 'sliding scale' principle – you have a set amount of insulin and glucose trickling into the bloodstream; if your blood glucose level starts to rise, the insulin is stepped up, and if it starts to fall, the insulin drip is slowed down. Talk to your obstetric team at the hospital where you hope to have the baby about their specific protocols for women with diabetes in labour.

Your blood glucose levels might start to fall during labour. This is, after all, the ultimate form of exercise. And, just as in a strenuous workout, you run the risk of going hypo. As soon as you have delivered the baby your insulin needs will drop dramatically – right down to your pre-pregnancy levels – so ask the team about their measures to prevent hypos during and after labour.

I have had Type 2 diabetes for five years, and my doctor just added a diagnosis of PCOS. Are they related?

Just as with Type 2 diabetes, polycystic ovary syndrome (PCOS) is characterized by insulin resistance. High cholesterol, hypertension and heart disease are also hallmark symptoms. PCOS triggers an overabundance of androgens (male sex hormones) and too little oestrogen, causing cysts to form in the ovaries.

Because of your diabetes, your labour and delivery team will be on the lookout for hypoglycaemia. While still in your womb, your baby's pancreas had been programmed to produce enough insulin to counteract your sometimes-heightened blood glucose supply. Once he becomes 'disconnected' from the maternal sugar source at delivery, his high insulin levels may drive his blood glucose down, causing hypoglycaemia. A heel prick blood test can confirm the diagnosis, and oral glucose or a glucose IV drip for the baby can quickly treat the condition.

Having a parent with Type 1 diabetes makes your child slightly more likely to develop the disease (2 to 5 per cent; higher if another parent or sibling has the disease). Type 2 has a stronger genetic link, but the good news is that it is easier to prevent with healthy lifestyle changes.

Breastfeeding

Many women with diabetes question their ability to breastfeed, worrying about either harm to their baby – Is my milk safe? Does it have enough nutrients? – or uncontrolled blood glucose swings in themselves –Will I go high from having to eat more? Will I go hypo from 'sharing' with my baby? You may be relieved to find out that women with diabetes can and do breastfeed successfully, and in fact your milk may even reduce the chances of your baby developing diabetes.

Breast Benefits

Babies who breastfeed for at least three months have a lower incidence of Type 1 diabetes, and may be less likely to become obese as adults. Some research has linked early exposure to cow's milk and cow's milk-based formula to the development of Type 1 diabetes – another good reason to nurse your child.

Clinical studies have also shown that women who have gestational diabetes in pregnancy and go on to breastfeed their child for at least three months experience improved pancreatic beta cell function, which may lessen their chances of developing Type 2 diabetes later. Breastfeeding may also be protective for the children of at-risk Type 2 populations.

Safety Measures

Taking insulin does not threaten the health of your breastfeeding infant. However, women who take medication to control Type 2 diabetes need to talk to their doctor, as some drugs pass into breastmilk. Your doctor can help you weigh the benefits of breastfeeding against any risks medication might pose – she may be able to prescribe an alternative drug. If you are pregnant and plan to breastfeed, you should discuss these issues with your doctor now, so you are both prepared once the baby arrives.

Breastfeeding can be hard work (especially for first-time mothers), and when you're trying to balance it with the demanding occupation of new motherhood, the stress and fatigue can affect your control. The hormonal changes associated with breastfeeding and the postpartum period can also cause highs and lows (although in some women, this shift may improve blood glucose levels). Checking your blood glucose levels often and working with your care team is the best way to stay on track.

As with mothers without diabetes, there is no set timetable for weaning. However, when you and your baby decide it is time, it should be done gradually if possible. In addition to stirring up the hormones again, you may have to adjust your diet to stay consistent with your control. Talk to your dietician about your particular needs.

Avoiding Hypos

You'll need extra calories and fluid in your daily diet to keep your milk supply and your energy level up. If you haven't seen your dietician lately, now's the time to go in for a refresher appointment. She can help you to create a meal plan that can promote successful breastfeeding, reasonable postpartum weight loss and good diabetes control.

Not surprisingly, nursing can cause a drop in blood glucose levels. To avoid this, have a protein/carbohydrate snack and something to drink either before or during nursing. This is particularly important for middle-of-the-night feedings. Keep quick and easy snacks to hand.

Glucose tablets or other fast-acting sugars should be easily accessible in case of a hypo, and a meter should be stowed within reach to make checking levels easy (but don't forget to store it more securely once your baby is old enough to get around, which will be sooner than you think).

When it's Time for Menopause

The big change usually brings about changes in your diabetes treatment needs as well. In addition to the mood swings, the slowdown of oestrogen and progesterone production can put your blood sugars on a swing of their own. In fact, you may start experiencing these symptoms before menopause, in the preceding period known as perimenopause, which starts anywhere from 45 to 55 (the average age being 47).

How Menopause Affects Diabetes

Lower oestrogen levels may increase insulin resistance in Type 2 women, while lower progesterone levels have the opposite effect, increasing insulin sensitivity. For this reason, one woman's blood glucose response to menopause can be very different from another's. The best way to find out what's going on with you is to test your glucose levels frequently and work closely with your doctor and diabetes specialist nurse.

The American Diabetes Association reports that most women require less medication (for blood glucose control) for Type 2 diabetes after menopause. However, weight gain, which occurs in response to a slowing metabolism and declining oestrogen levels, may offset this benefit, as can inactivity. Postmenopausal women with diabetes have a risk of heart attack or stroke that is up to three times that of their peers without diabetes. This is because women with diabetes don't seem to have the natural premenopausal protection against heart disease and stroke that women without diabetes have.

HRT: Risks Versus Benefits

Whether or not to take hormone replacement therapy to combat some of the menopausal problems unique to women with diabetes is an individual decision, based on your own medical situation and cardio-vascular risk profile. Oral oestrogen therapy may improve your cholesterol profile by lowering your LDL (bad) and raising your HDL (good) cholesterol, but it has also been found to increase triglyceride levels, which ups cardiovascular risk.Preliminary data released in 2002 by the US Women's Health Initiative trial found that HRT oestrogen/progestogen therapy increased the risk of breast cancer, pulmonary embolism and cardiovascular disease in postmenopausal women. It's unclear whether oestrogen therapy alone carries similar health risks.

Female Sexual Dysfunction

In this post-Viagra age, the British public is well aware of the problems of male impotency. But female sexual dysfunction and arousal problems remain a less publicized cause. However, according to results of a national study published in the *Journal of the American Medical Association* in 1999, sexual dysfunction was actually more prevalent in women than in men (43 as opposed to 31 per cent).

If you're suffering from sexual dysfunction, you need to talk to your GP about the problem. In some cases, it may be a sign of an underlying, undiagnosed diabetic complication that needs treatment. Even if it is something more benign, you owe it to yourself to find a solution. Don't let embarrassment stop you – your doctor is there to help.

Uncontrolled blood glucose levels affect arousal, performance and overall well-being. High blood glucose levels trigger yeast infections and vaginal irritation. In addition, vascular damage can restrict blood flow to the vagina, causing lubrication problems. Women who have neuropathy that affects the genital area, the reproductive organs and/or the vagina may have difficulty achieving arousal and orgasm.

Psychological Factors

Sometimes the problem is more psychological than physical. The less-romantic aspects of treatment, such as needing to do a blood glucose check before sex, can make some women self-conscious and less likely to initiate or participate in it.

Fear may be a factor in your ability to let go and relax, as well. You may be afraid that the physical exertion of sex will trigger hypoglycaemia. Taking the same precautions as for exercise will almost always prevent low blood sugar levels. However, make sure your partner knows that in the unlikely event that you do lose consciousness, it wasn't his performance that did it. Give him a briefing on when to seek emergency medical care for you. Chapter 14 has more on hypoglycaemia prevention and education.

Other Culprits

A number of other issues can contribute to sexual difficulties in women with diabetes. These include:

· Certain medications (antidepressants, hypertension medications)
· Menopause (low oestrogen levels can cause vaginal dryness)
· Vaginismus (a tightening of the vaginal walls that may make sex painful)
· Excess weight or obesity – women who are overweight may feel self-conscious and unattractive.

Wearing an insulin pump can present some unique challenges in the bedroom. If you decide you want to disconnect it before sex, make sure you take into account the amount of time you are off the pump and the exertion factor, and adjust accordingly once you're connected again. If you prefer to stay hooked up, you may choose to use a longer infusion or tubing set.

Treatments

Therapy and/or medication may help you overcome depression. Make sure you talk to your doctor about the possible sexual side effects of any antidepressant she may prescribe.

If low oestrogen levels are at the root of vaginal dryness problems, vaginal oestrogen cream can sometimes alleviate this problem, but it should be prescribed with caution in some women. Over-the-counter lubricants are also available to ease dryness and painful penetration. Medical devices designed to stimulate blood flow in the genitals and increase lubrication may also be prescribed. Your GP can tell you more about these options, and may refer you to a gynaecologist if necessary.

As with most complications related to diabetes, adjustments to your diet, medication and exercise routines may improve both your diabetes and your sex drive.

How Women Cope

Managing chronic illness day in and day out can be stressful and emotionally draining. If you have been diagnosed recently, you're trying to get your mental and physical bearings to find out your own path to diabetes control. You've been thrown into this disease headfirst and, even with the best diabetes care team guiding you, these early days can be stressful, scary and anxious. In a worst-case scenario, you may have been handed a diagnosis, a one-size-fits-all 'diabetic diet' and/or prescription, and shown the door to work things out on your own.

Dealing With Depression

People with diabetes are up to three times more likely to suffer from depression than the general population, and women with diabetes are more likely to experience depression than men with the disease. It's normal to experience some depressive symptoms when diabetes is diagnosed, but when depression starts to interfere with everyday life and you start to lose interest in things you used to enjoy, you may be experiencing a major depressive episode.

Depression distracts you from proper diabetes care, and clinical studies have shown that people with diabetes who are depressed have higher blood glucose levels and a higher incidence of microvascular and macrovascular diabetic complications. Add poor control, and the symptoms and psychological impact of knowing you aren't doing well with your diabetes care can make you even more depressed, resulting in a downward spiral of blood glucose highs and emotional lows.

Diabetes can be a heavy load to carry, and depression seems to double that weight. Ignore either and they'll only get worse. You don't have to suffer in silence. Let your doctor know if you're experiencing signs of depression. Counselling or antidepressant medication may be options for you to explore.

Weighty Issues

Women with Type 1 diabetes may find their weight fluctuating with their insulin needs, which can be a source of frustration and may also take a toll on self-esteem, particularly in the teenage years. For women with Type 2 diabetes, who often have weight problems, negative body image is a prevalent problem.

Apart from contributing to depression, a poor self-image can hinder your sex life and be a source of stress and anxiety. Living a fit and active lifestyle should not be identified with being supermodel-skinny. Accepting yourself – at any size – is important to your physical and psychological well-being.

Sometimes weight problems can feel so insurmountable that women hesitate to even take that first step forwards for fear of failure. Soon they find themselves in an endless cycle of binging, bad feelings and sky-high blood glucose levels. Consequently, self-esteem plummets along with diabetes control. Yes, weight loss can be hard, but you don't have to go it alone. Your doctor, dietician and diabetes specialist nurse are all there to help you succeed. See Chapter 13 for more information on the psychology of weight loss and sensible weight control.

Chapter 19

Special Issues for Men

Men with diabetes face unique challenges of their own. You may be less apt to express any feelings of anxiety or depression you're facing while trying to come to terms with the disease, and one of the most prevalent complications in men with diabetes – impotence – is definitely an emotionally loaded issue. But while men face a higher risk of certain diabetic complications, they are more likely to report feeling in control of their diabetes and on top of their treatment – both of benefit when dealing with chronic disease.

At Puberty

The peak incidence of Type 1 diabetes in boys is between the ages of 12 and 14, when puberty is up and running. The hormonal changes that accompany puberty actually increase insulin resistance in both boys and girls, which compounds the problem of insufficient insulin production in those with Type 1 diabetes.

Additionally, insulin resistance may also be accompanied by increased resistance to growth hormone in boys, and poor control has the potential to impact the speed and course of the 'growth spurt' that normally occurs at puberty.

A Turbulent Time

Puberty is a time of separation from parents and a growing emphasis on social relationships – creating a separate social identity is paramount. Boys who may have depended on their parents for guidance on diabetes care may start taking more responsibility for their care. Similarly, parents must learn to hand over the reins of diabetes control, at least partially, to allow their child to mature emotionally as well as physically.

However, the social pressures of puberty can also push young men in the opposite direction, that of ignoring their diabetes for the sake of being more like their peers. Drug and alcohol use – experimental or otherwise – can also become a problem during this time of life.

Because alcohol can impair treatment judgment and trigger a potentially dangerous hypoglycaemic episode, it's important that boys (and girls) with diabetes are educated about the special risks they face with alcohol and drug use. Even though 'Just Say No' may be good advice, realistically, it may not be followed. Especially during adolescence, kids need to know what precautions are necessary if they do drink.

Changes in Testosterone Levels

Testosterone levels in men begin to decrease starting around the age of 40, eventually leading to what some have called the 'male menopause', or andropause, which brings with it an increased cardiovascular risk, loss of muscle and bone mass and a waning libido. Other signs of declining testosterone can include lower sperm count, body hair loss, and even episodes of hot flushes.

tips

While low levels of testosterone are thought to be associated with central obesity, the opposite is true for women, in whom high levels of the hormone are tied to excess abdominal fat and insulin resistance.

Men with diabetes tend to have a lower than average testosterone level. The classic 'apple-shaped' body of Type 2 diabetes, also known variously as intra-abdominal fat or central fat storage (or, in more familiar terms, beer belly), is associated with low testosterone levels in men. Also known as hypogonadism, this condition is also associated with high levels of circulating insulin (hyperinsulinaemia) and increased insulin resistance. Low levels of the hormone are thought to affect glucose metabolism; some studies have linked improved glucose tolerance with testosterone replacement therapy.

HRT – Not Just for Women

Hormone replacement therapy, in the form of injections or a transdermal (through the skin) gel or patch, can be beneficial to many older men with low testosterone levels. The jury is still out on whether this therapy can slow or even prevent the onset of Type 2 diabetes by inhibiting intra-abdominal fat accumulation.

Sexuality and Impotence

Impotence – the failure to achieve or maintain an erection – is one of the most common and most distressing side effects of diabetes. Overall, about 35 per cent of men with diabetes suffer from impotence (known as 'erectile dysfunction' or sometimes ED in medical terminology), and this figure rises to over 50 per cent of men over the age of 50. If you've experienced problems with impotence, then take heart because you're by no means alone.

Some men delay searching for treatment for impotence because of embarrassment or self-consciousness, but impotence can be the first sign of a more serious underlying diabetes complication, such as cardiovascular disease or neuropathy, so it's important not to ignore it or to delay medical attention for the problem. Your doctor will be quite used to dealing with impotence issues and will have a variety of treatment options at his disposal.

What Causes Impotence

There are many possible causes of male impotence, ranging from complications after surgery to smoking; the following are most likely to affect men with diabetes:

- **Medications.** Drugs such as high blood pressure medications, certain antidepressants and tranquillizers can trigger episodes of impotence. Your doctor may be able to adjust your dosage or substitute another medication.
- **Neuropathy.** Nerve damage to the penis itself or to the autonomic nervous system may be the cause of impotence.
- **Cardiovascular disease.** Clogged arteries, especially those that feed the corpora cavernosa (the spongy vascular tissue of the penis) can impair circulation enough to inhibit an erection and thus lead to impotence.
- **Psychological issues.** Depression, anxiety and stress related to diabetes management can inhibit sexual performance.

Smoking can contribute to erectile dysfunction by causing constriction of the blood vessels, leading to hypertension. Nicotine also promotes the growth of artery-clogging cholesterol plaques, which also contribute to high blood pressure.

Treatment Options

There are a number of options available for treating impotence, including medication, vacuum devices, surgery and psychosocial therapy. The least-invasive non-pharmaceutical method of treatment is a mechanical vacuum device. A cylinder is placed over the length of the penis and a hand-operated vacuum pump is used to remove the air from the cylinder, creating a vacuum and pulling blood into the penis to create an erection. Once erection has been achieved, it is sustained with the use of a tension ring placed at the base of the penis.

The thought of a hypodermic syringe anywhere near your groin area might send shivers down your spine, but many men with impotence caused by neuropathy can be helped with drugs that are injected directly into the penis to dilate, or widen, blood vessels and cause an erection. Alprostadil is available in injectable form (Caverject or Viridal Duo) and also as a suppository that can be inserted into the urethra (MUSE), a more palatable choice for some men.

Viagra (sildenafil) is well known and has helped many men with erectile dysfunction problems since it officially became available in the UK in 1999. The drug is taken about an hour before sexual activity and works by enhancing the effects of nitric oxide on the body, which dilates blood vessels and acts as a smooth-muscle relaxant. This improves blood flow to the penis and facilitates an erection when sexual arousal occurs.

Several clinical studies have demonstrated that Viagra is well-tolerated by men with both Type 1 and Type 2 diabetes, and can help these men improve their erectile function significantly. One potential drawback is the need to take the drug 60 minutes before sex; if you're a spur-of-the-moment type, you'll need a new strategy.

Two new drugs for erectile dysfunction are now available in the UK: Tadalafil (Cialis) and vardenafil (Levitra) work in the same way as sildenafil (Viagra).

All three oral drugs used to treat erectile dysfunction are available free on the NHS to men with diabetes. However, free prescription is limited to four tablets per month; if you want more, then you may have to get a private prescription and pay the doctor and dispensing pharmacy. Diabetes UK strongly recommends that people do not purchase these drugs over the Internet or by mail order – it is crucial that you consult your doctor before taking them in case they are not appropriate for you.

Men taking nitrates in any medications must not take Viagra, Cialis or Levitra because a large and sudden drop in blood pressure may occur. Nitrates include the heart medicine glyceryl trinitrate (GTN) commonly used to treat angina.

Insertion of a penile implant, or treatment and repair of arterial and venous damage related to impotence, are more invasive options for treating impotence. Your doctor can discuss treatment options that are right for you.

If your impotence is rooted in depression, anxiety or other emotional issues, your doctor may refer you to a counsellor, psychiatrist or psychologist for help in sorting through it all. A Relate counsellor may also be helpful for uncovering sources of marital tension.

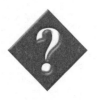

I have diabetes and hypertension. Can sex make my heart condition worse?
Unless your heart is severely impaired (i.e. congestive heart failure), there is really very little risk of normal sexual activity triggering a heart attack. Halting all exercise – and sex – is probably one of the worst things for your hypertension. A chat with your doctor about your concerns will help you ease your mind about sex.

Diabetes and Fertility

Men with long-term, uncontrolled diabetes can suffer nerve damage that causes a condition known as *retrograde ejaculation*, where sperm is deposited into the urinary bladder instead of being ejaculated from the head of the penis. This happens because the small muscle that controls the passageway into the bladder becomes damaged and doesn't close as it should during climax, so sperm is re-routed into the bladder.

Some men may have reduced ejaculate as a result of this condition, while others may not ejaculate at all. The latter is referred to as 'dry climax'. Retrograde ejaculation can be a cause of male infertility, and if it is caused by neuropathy it cannot be surgically corrected at this point in time.

If you have symptoms of the condition, you should talk to your doctor about a referral to a urologist. Couples who have trouble conceiving due to retrograde ejaculation should see a fertility specialist. Assisted reproduction may be a possibility by retrieving sperm through a bladder-washing procedure and using it for artificial insemination.

Complications: Gender Bias?

While diabetes crosses all age, racial and gender lines, it does seem to show some questionably preferential treatment to men in the distribution of certain diabetic complications. For example, it is reported that men diagnosed with diabetes before the age of 30 tend to develop retinopathy more rapidly than their female counterparts. Among people with diabetes, first heart attacks are more likely to be fatal in men than women.

f(a)ct Amputation rates are reportedly 1.4–2.7 times higher in men than in women, according to the American Diabetes Association. However, with preventative foot care and wound treatment, your risk drops dramatically.

Men with Type 2 diabetes are more likely to develop coronary artery disease (CAD) than women with the disease and than their male counterparts without diabetes. They are also more likely to have additional CAD risk factors, such as high triglycerides, high blood pressure and obesity.

How Men Cope

A ten-year study of gender differences in attitudes towards diabetes at the Johns Hopkins Diabetes Centre in the USA found that men tended to have more positive attitudes towards, and greater acceptance of, their diabetes than women with the disease. Accordingly, they also tended to rate their quality of life higher. The study also found that men were more accepting of their treatment regime, and were less likely to miss work or leisure activities due to their diabetes.

Perhaps reflecting traditional gender roles, men with diabetes were also most satisfied with the level of emotional support they received from their partners, who were more likely to accompany them to appointments and diabetes education classes than male partners of women with diabetes. Interestingly, while men with diabetes did not miss work or leisure activities, their wives were more likely to have to take time off attributed to their husband's disease, yet these women reported feeling less anxious about the long-term impact of the disease on their family than the husbands of women with diabetes.

Men in this study also reported more control over their diabetes in terms of lower HbA1c levels, better self-reported nutritional care and insulin compliance, and fewer complications than the women.

Men and Stress Management

But what about when things don't go right? Problems with erratic blood glucose levels and elusive control can cause stress levels to climb; high stress then produces high glucose levels, high blood pressure, and further anxiety about your ability to manage your disease.

When things aren't going well with diabetes management, some men can take it as a sign of personal failure, or an affront to their masculinity, and the resulting stress can make the situation worse. Think of erratic blood glucose levels as a challenge rather than a fault. Use your health care team and your support system to figure out the mystery.

Studies have demonstrated that stress management training can improve long-term blood glucose control, reducing your risk of complications. They have also demonstrated that daily practice of stress-management techniques by men with heart disease can slash their risk of cardiovascular incidents such as surgery and heart attack.

Chapter 20

Diabetes, Emotions and Relationships

In addition to blood glucose highs and lows, diabetes triggers emotional ups and downs that can be just as unpredictable and severe. And because the disease is life-altering, it has a significant impact not just on the patient, but on everyone who lives with and cares for her or him. Preparing yourself for the emotional issues that diabetes brings can help you maintain your sanity and strengthen your relationships with others.

Dealing With Diagnosis

Dealing with a diabetes diagnosis has been compared to coping with the grief of death. Diagnosis marks the loss of life as you knew it. It's normal to grieve for your old 'healthy' life, even if you weren't feeling well before getting the diabetes label. Denial, anger, bargaining, depression and acceptance are all part of the process.

The Dangers of Denial

The first of these can be the hardest and most damaging in diabetes. Many people choose to simply ignore that they have the disease, continuing as if it didn't exist. The problem with this (non)coping approach is the long-term consequences of uncontrolled blood glucose. By the time people do come to terms with denial and are ready to treat their diabetes, serious complications may be on their way.

Some newly diagnosed patients will acknowledge their feelings of denial. Recognition is a good sign that in the back of your mind you know you must move forward. As long as you're willing to follow your doctor's orders for the time being, even if you haven't fully accepted the disease, denial is a normal part of the process.

For patients who reject both the diagnosis and the treatment, the situation can become a dangerous one. Sometimes it takes a blood glucose emergency that lands them in hospital for them to realize that they do, indeed, have diabetes.

Reaching acceptance can be a difficult, rocky road. Many people need the help of a therapist or counsellor to get there. A health psychologist who has specialized training in the intricate psychological, biological and social relationships between physical illness and mental health can be helpful in sorting through coping issues.

The Emotional Roller Coaster

Although acceptance is an important step in getting on track to diabetes control, it isn't a guarantee of ongoing inner peace. Periods of difficult control and high blood glucose levels can also bring devastating emotional lows, which can in turn make blood glucose levels rise even further and start a self-perpetuating cycle of physical and psychological deterioration. Learn to recognize the signs of emotional pitfalls such as depression, anger, guilt and stress, so you can take the appropriate steps to stop this downward spiral before it starts.

Depression

Studies suggest that 15–20 per cent of people with diabetes also suffer from a major depressive disorder. Researchers analyzing numerous studies have reported that the risk of major depressive disorders is more than doubled in people with diabetes. Occasional sadness, fear and uncertainty are normal in diabetes, but when they start affecting your everyday enjoyment of life and interfering with proper self-care, they may be something more than just a passing emotional downturn.

Signs of a depressive disorder include weight loss, insomnia or hypersomnia (too little or too much sleep), irritability or agitation, fatigue, feelings of guilt or worthlessness, inability to concentrate and recurrent thoughts of death or suicide.

Depression can be treated with therapy and/or antidepressant medication, so there's no reason to suffer needlessly. Here are a few strategies that may help you deal with depression:

· **Knowledge is power.** Fear of the unknown can feed your depression. If you haven't already, start educating yourself about your disease.
· **Seek support.** Draw on the experience and emotional comfort of your family, friends, spiritual community, health care team and others with diabetes.

- **Keep perfection in perspective.** Reward your successes, big or small, and try to see your stumbles as learning experiences, not failures.
- **Keep moving.** Try to push yourself to at least take a brisk walk daily. Exercise raises your endorphin levels, a natural mood booster.

Anger Management

You have diabetes and you're foot-stamping, wall-slamming, steaming mad about it. Now what do you do with all that pent-up hostility? Do you focus it on beating the daylights out of that damn disease through aggressive diabetes control, or do you turn it out at the world and push away your family and care providers in the process?

Anger is an understandable reaction to diabetes, and it can be a good motivational tool if used appropriately. However, if it's becoming a barrier to your care and your relationships with others, it's a problem.

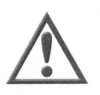

Anger is a common symptom of low blood glucose. If you feel yourself getting angry for no good reason, it may be a sign you need to test your blood glucose. If you live with someone with diabetes, try not to take anger personally when it occurs in connection with a hypo. Remind yourself that it's the diabetes talking, and concentrate on treating the hypoglycaemia.

Feeling Guilty

It may not be rational, but it's perfectly normal to feel guilty about having diabetes. But now that you know it's normal, it's time to move on. You are not to blame for having diabetes, nor should you feel ashamed of your diagnosis. You've done nothing to deserve your disease; your genetic make-up and/or environmental factors have made you susceptible to it through no fault of your own.

Managing Stress

When you face a physically or psychologically stressful situation, your body starts a complex process of hormone release and reaction. The adrenal glands start to pump out cortisol, the hormone primarily responsible for our physiological 'fight or flight' reaction to situations we perceive as dangerous. Cortisol signals the liver to start up glucose production to give the brain and central nervous system added energy, while signalling to the fat and muscle tissues to slow their uptake. It also causes the release of fatty acids from fat tissues, which are needed for muscle fuel, and sends your blood pressure up.

No one, and that means no one, has perfect diabetes management skills all the time. If you have an unforeseen high or low, don't take it as a sign of personal failure. Measure your success by your commitment to care. When a high or low happens, learn from the experience to prevent it the next time.

Stress also prompts the adrenal glands to release adrenaline, the hormone that provides the adrenaline rush of the 'fight or flight' reaction. High levels of circulating cortisol and adrenaline promote insulin resistance in addition to cranking up blood glucose levels.

Since it increases blood pressure and raises glucose levels, stress is obviously not the best medicine for diabetes control. And it's dangerous because it may distract you from controlling your diabetes as you become preoccupied with other issues.

The Physical Toll

When you're ill or suffer an injury, your body is stressed and you need to test more frequently. The same goes for times when you are mentally and emotionally under duress. Sorting out your Income Tax returns? On double shifts at work? Taking final exams? Make sure you test glucose levels more often than usual.

Stress has also been associated with abdominal or visceral adiposity (that 'apple' shape); it's unclear, though, whether stress causes a spare tyre and the spare tyre causes Type 2.

Make a Change

Studies have shown that stress-management programmes can be extremely effective in improving psychological well-being and diabetes control. One 2002 US study, published in *Diabetes Care*, found that just five sessions of stress management training lowered HbA1c levels an average of half a percentage point. The study involved a stress-training regime of progressive muscle relaxation, cognitive and behavioural therapy (including guided imagery and deep-breathing exercises), and education on the mechanisms and health consequences of stress.

Other good stress-management techniques include yoga, music or art therapy, and writing a journal. Anything that calms you and allows you to relax and release is a good stress-management strategy.

Turning to a Support Group

Support groups are an invaluable resource, offering patients a chance to compare treatment notes, to talk about emotional issues in living with the disease – even to moan about the health care system. In addition to expanding your knowledge and fostering a sense of camaraderie, a support group is a good stress-release valve.

You can find out about local diabetes groups from your doctor's surgery or local hospital. Diabetes UK has a large number of voluntary groups across the UK; some function mainly as fund-raising groups, others as support or self-help groups. Ask your doctor or diabetes nurse about the possible interest level in a group among other patients. You may even be able to set up one of your own; contact the Voluntary Groups section of Diabetes UK (see Appendix A) for guidance on how to go about setting up a group.

While physical stress causes blood glucose levels to rise in both Type 1 and Type 2, mental stress consistently causes rises only in Type 2 diabetes. Most people with Type 1 diabetes will also have a rise in levels in conjunction with psychological stress, but some will experience a drop.

Around the World

Online communities for people with diabetes are plentiful and can be almost as – if not more – supportive and informative than real-time groups. There's input from Peterborough to Pittsburgh, with participants from all walks of life and a broad range of experience with diabetes and diabetic complications. On the other hand, you may get inaccurate medical information from people who either don't know better or who are trying to sell some miracle cure.

The 'miracle' workers can be taken care of with the firm hand of a good moderator. As long as you take what you read with a pinch of salt, you certainly stand more to gain than you can lose. And the beauty of an online support group is that it is there all day and all night for your questions, thoughts and problems.

The Dating Game

Single with diabetes? You may feel like every encounter is a blind date as you consider whether or not to 'tell' about your diabetes. Or you may screen your potential partners by specifically mentioning the 'D' word. There's no reason to treat your diabetes as a skeleton in the closet or a secret, but some people feel more comfortable sharing their disease after they've laid the foundation for a relationship. Do what feels right for you.

Intimacy Issues

When things get intimate, they can also get a little weird. What if you go hypo and pass out in the heat of passion? Or what if your partner gets tangled up in your insulin pump infusion set? Having a sexual encounter of the strange kind is the worst nightmare of many single people living with diabetes.

Making love with a partner you trust can alleviate much of the tension you might feel about your first time together. What seems mortifying now is usually good for a laugh together later. The worst-case scenario rarely happens. Don't obsess over the 'coulds' to the point where they become a major preoccupation.

For Spouses and Partners

When your partner is handed a diabetes diagnosis, so are you. Get on board with diabetes care right away. You can and should attend diabetes education classes to learn more about the disease and how to treat it. If you do the food shopping and/or cooking in your household, you should absolutely attend the meetings your partner has with a dietician. If your partner feels comfortable with it, go along on doctor's visits as well. Two sets of ears are always better than one.

My husband has had problems in the bedroom ever since he was diagnosed with Type 2 diabetes. Is this part of the disease?
If your husband is newly diagnosed, he may be struggling to come to terms with diabetes. Depression, anxiety and anger are all common emotions following diagnosis of a chronic illness, and could temporarily affect his libido. However, diabetes-associated impotence is quite common. For more on the subject, see Chapter 19.

Try (and it can be hard) not to become the diabetes patrol. Think of what it would be like to go through life listening to the following:

· 'Are you sure you can eat that?'
· 'Do you *really* think you should have that?'
· 'Don't you think you should do something about that reading?'

Communicate openly and honestly with your partner about how you can help when things aren't going right, before they go astray. That way you know in advance the most effective way to assist.

Helping Those Who Don't Help Themselves

Perhaps you're reading this book because you're more interested in diabetes control than your partner – the one with the disease – is. Maybe your partner hasn't come to terms with his diagnosis yet, or maybe he's depressed or disheartened and has stopped trying. You can read and learn until you're blue in the face, and you may even be able to persuade your partner into a few extra glucose checks or a more appropriate meal. But you can't control his diabetes for him. Remember this if you remember nothing else. Your mental health and emotional well-being are just as important as your partner's, and you can save yourself countless hours of head-banging frustration if you can be detached enough to realize that he is the pilot of the diabetes ship.

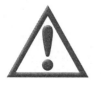

> Support your spouse or partner, but keep in mind that she, and not you, is in charge of taking care of her diabetes. This means being there for her if she asks for help, offering to go to the doctor's appointments with her, but not pushing the issue, and not eating things under her nose that she would love to have but shouldn't.

At the same time, you don't want to go too far in the other direction and make it easier for your partner to get away with messing up his control by going along with his programme. Accepting his excuses about why that extra piece of pie just had to be eaten, or nodding your head when she says she's going to cut back her insulin to lose some weight is not being supportive. It's called 'enabling', and spouses and family members of alcoholics do it all the time. Don't let yourself become part of the problem, or validate bad behaviour.

Caring for Kids With Diabetes

Diabetes affects the entire family – beyond the lifestyle adjustments a family is faced with, there are fear, guilt, jealousy, anger and other emotions to come to terms with. Both the parent/child and the sibling relationship can face difficult challenges that require empathy, discipline and flexibility to work through and beyond.

Whether a parent or child has diabetes, the whole family can benefit from diabetes education classes. Even small children can learn more about the disease through age-appropriate books. It's easy to feel isolated when you have diabetes, and involving the family goes a long way towards creating a caring and supportive environment that makes control easier.

To Love and Not Overprotect

When your child has diabetes, he or she has more boundaries than others, and it can be easy to fall into the trap of making them tighter than necessary. Letting your fears overtake your child's normal social development is not healthy for either of you. Kids need to be kids – to participate in sports, to go to birthday parties, to spend the day at the beach with friends, and to go to dances and football matches.

Follow the 'first do no harm' motto of the medical profession and take the least invasive route when making decisions on what your child can and cannot do, based on your child's age, responsibility and level of competence with her or his own diabetes care. And if you must say no, let your child know the reasoning behind the decision. 'Because I said so' is not a good explanation, and will not help to make boundaries clearer to your son or daughter.

As your child grows and takes greater control over her own care, you may find yourself feeling strangely unneeded. Remember that your adolescent is forming her own identity and needs the autonomy to make some of her own treatment decisions and take over more of her day-to-day management. You do need to remain a partner in her care, however. Asking if she's changed her infusion set or helping her check her glucose if she doesn't look well is still your responsibility as parent and care partner.

Sibling Issues

One child has diabetes and the other doesn't. How do you balance one child's restrictions with the other's relative lack of them? How do you balance out all the necessary time and attention given to caring for your child with diabetes in the eyes of your child who doesn't require constant oversight? Parenting can be even more of a challenge when you're caring for a child with diabetes and a child without it. You feel as if you're constantly saying 'no' to both of them.

Caregivers need care, too. While it becomes easier with practice and age, it's emotionally exhausting to stand guard over your child day in and day out. Arrange for back-up care for your child at least once a month, and get out and enjoy yourself. You might also check the availability of support groups for parents of children with diabetes in your area, as both a sounding board and a shoulder to lean on.

Try to make life as normal as possible for both of them. Healthy eating habits and activity should be a family goal. The sibling without diabetes should be educated about the other's special needs, something that will probably come naturally in the course of everyday home life. However, you need to make it clear that only parents or another responsible adult are to treat the disease, as some children may try to 'help' with a younger sibling and unknowingly place them in danger. Your child with diabetes needs to feel safe about his care, and also guilt-free about having special requirements associated with the disease.

At the same time, don't let your child get manipulative with his disease. Using it as an excuse to get out of chores or tasks, or playing the 'poor me' card to get you to agree to special privileges should not be allowed, particularly when it's at the expense of your other child. Being a parent of a dual-diagnosis (one with, one without) household can be a challenge, but you're up to the task. To learn more about parenting a child with diabetes, see Chapter 17.

Chapter 21

Living Life With Diabetes

In theory, there's almost nothing you can't do now that you couldn't do before you had diabetes. But in practice, you will have to make some lifestyle adjustments to manage your disease well. It's like the old joke – 'Doctor, will I ever be able to play the violin again? Yes? That's great – I couldn't play it before...' You may actually be able to do things bigger and better than you could before your diagnosis.

Diabetes at Home

Even though you're the one with the diabetes diagnosis, your whole family needs to make some adjustments to living with the disease. A healthy lifestyle promoting good blood glucose control is the best defence against diabetic complications. And the good news is that it's a great prescription for everyone around you as well.

Don't try to go it alone. The changes that diabetes brings to the dinner table can be positive ones for the entire family, particularly if your diet before now has been less than stellar. Exercise is also a healthy choice for the whole family, both physically and on a psychological level – the family that plays together stays together.

While kids should be able to enjoy the occasional treat that isn't regularly on your meal plan, stocking up on junk food isn't healthy for you or them. You don't need the temptation – and they will be better off with more balanced fare. Limit 'treats' to special occasions such as Christmas or birthdays.

You may hear the 'why should we all have to suffer?' defence as you encourage your family to join you on your new and healthier lifestyle. Step back and assess what might be causing that reaction. Fear of giving up the familiar is one possibility. You might also be asking them to do too much too fast, particularly if you were stuck in a pizza, Chinese takeaway and McDonald's routine.

Start Out Slowly

Try limiting restaurant food to once a week and encouraging healthier menu choices. Instead of declaring 'no junk food' all at once, allow one selection of their choosing to be kept in a cabinet you don't use. Above all, work to provide lots of healthy, fresh and good-tasting alternatives so the change is perceived as a positive one.

If your family members have a favourite food that's no longer for you, only keep it around if you're sure it won't be calling you from the larder.

Remember, you are not an ogre for requesting that crisps, cakes and chocolate bars be kept out of the kitchen. No matter what degree of pouting and resistance you face from your spouse or children, stand firm. Bypassing these treats won't harm their health; having them could very well hurt yours.

Make Your Needs Known

It's easy to get discouraged and depressed when others don't seem to be meeting your needs or don't even seem to be aware that you have them. Stop those feelings before they start by laying out exactly what you need from the people around you.

If you find you don't have enough time to exercise as you should because of child care responsibilities, tell your spouse it's essential to your health to get some assistance. If your partner keeps making you all the things you shouldn't be eating, give her some guidance. Go with her on the next shopping expedition, or, better, take her with you on your next appointment with your doctor, diabetes nurse or dietician. Don't expect your family and friends to be mind-readers. Assume they know next to nothing about your new lifestyle needs, and educate them accordingly.

Making Your Home Diabetes-Friendly

There's more to treatment success than whipping the kitchen into shape. The first is keeping a frequent watch on where your glucose levels are. One way to encourage yourself is to have several meters available where you'll use them – in the kitchen, by your bed, in your sports bag. If you're often testing at night, there's at least one model on the market with a glow-in-the-dark faceplate for easier testing. You can use your kitchen timer or alarm clock to remind you to take any postprandial blood glucose checks. Keep several blood glucose logs with your meters so you remember to record your results, or carry a pocket-sized 'master log' with you to keep everything in one place.

Home safety is also an issue. If you don't have one already, get a sharps disposal bin. Even if you don't use insulin, you should still have one for your lancets. If you have a small child with Type 1 diabetes, you will have to be twice as vigilant about toddler-proofing your home, particularly the kitchen. Keep the cupboards and larder closed and locked (or fastened with child safety latches) to avoid any surreptitious snacking.

Stress is a well-known offender in causing blood glucose levels to rise, particularly in patients with Type 2 diabetes. Yoga, progressive relaxation, massage therapy, exercise and meditation are just a few ways to de-stress. Talk therapy, either one-to-one with a counsellor or in a support group, can also be extremely helpful.

Diabetes at Work

If you are employed outside the home, you may need to make some adjustments in your daily work routine to accommodate good treatment habits. There's probably no job out there that is perfectly suited for diabetes, but there are some employment situations that are more difficult than others. Working a job where you're on your feet all day, where it's difficult to take a break to test your blood glucose, where your shifts are unpredictable or where you are exposed to extreme heat or cold can make control hard.

You may be faced with some hard choices as you try to make your job compatible with your new life. The legal protections offered by the Disability Discrimination Act (1995) will help to a degree, but even with that, you may find yourself in a position where your job is working against your diabetes management. If this is the case, you do have options:

- Talk to your doctor about adjustments to your treatment. Could a new medication or insulin regime help?
- Talk to your boss or manager about adjustments to your work schedule or other accommodations. Is a transfer possible or preferred? Could a shift change be in order?
- Explore your options both inside and outside your company. If you've been contemplating a career change or further education, maybe now is the time to get moving.

Shift work where your work shifts are switched on a regular basis is particularly hard on diabetes management, which strives for balance. If you must work these types of hours, you need to stay in close contact with your diabetes care team to keep on top of problems as they arise and make any necessary medication and insulin adjustments.

Discrimination: What the Law Says

The Disability Discrimination Act (DDA) defines disability as 'physical or mental impairment which has a substantial and long-term effect on a person's ability to carry out normal day-to-day activities'. Progressive conditions – such as diabetes – where symptoms would satisfy the Act's requirements if medication was not taken, are covered by the legislation. The act prevents your employer from treating you less favourably on account of having diabetes, and it requires that your employer makes 'reasonable adjustments', for example to allow you to check your blood glucose and treat yourself as needed (by having a snack).

I don't consider myself disabled just because I have diabetes. Am I sending the wrong message to my employer and colleagues if I claim protection under the DDA?
The DDA was designed to cover a broad range of people who may experience discrimination in the workplace due to health issues, and is your best protection for fair treatment on the job. Don't toss it aside based on semantics alone. When you invoke your rights under the DDA, you ensure you are judged on your abilities rather than your disease.

Giving you short breaks to check glucose, and adjusting your work shift if it causes control problems would fall under the scope of reasonable adjustments in most cases. However, if the adjustments are considered not justifiable (usually on the grounds of financial resources) then the requested steps may not be taken. Generally speaking, the majority of adjustments that would be required for diabetes would not be considered an undue hardship under the DDA for most organizations.

Job Hunting

Looking for a job? The DDA protects you against discrimination here as well. Prospective employers must be careful not to discriminate against people with diabetes in the following ways:

· How they decide who gets the job; how applications are handled or the interview carried out
· The terms on which they offer a job – for example, only giving a short-term contract
· By not offering the job.

If your diabetes is disclosed during a pre-employment health check, your prospective employer cannot use it as a reason to deny you employment as long as reasonable accommodations can be made for you. Of course, going for the head wine-taster job at the local vineyard isn't a good idea; there may be certain positions that require activities you just can't perform or that can't be reasonably accommodated. However, if you already are in one of these positions and develop diabetes, your employer must offer you another suitable vacant position within the company (as long as you are qualified to perform the new job). The DDA also prevents your employer from denying you a promotion based on your diabetes.

If, based on the employer's words or actions, you have any reason to believe you have been discriminated against because of your disease, you can call the Disability Rights Commission Helpline (Monday to Friday 8am–8pm), on 0845 7622 633.

Workplace Accommodations

There are many benefits to providing a working environment that accommodates people with diabetes and other chronic illnesses. Employee satisfaction, better attendance and staying in the job for longer, fewer sick days and lower disability payout are just a few good motivations. It also takes money and resources to train employees, and if you are a good worker, it makes sense for your employer to do what it can to retain you.

If the people in your workplace don't seem to know a lot about diabetes, take the opportunity to teach them.

To Tell or Not to Tell

Telling others about your diabetes can be particularly hard. You may be afraid of job discrimination. Sometimes it can be difficult admitting that you need help. However, you can't claim protection under the DDA if you don't let your employer know about your condition and ask for adjustment assistance. If you're inexplicably missing work or taking longer or more frequent breaks without permission, you may very well lose your job.

In addition to all the above reasons, there are several good reasons to let your colleagues in on your diabetes. First and foremost, people around you need to know what to do in case of a blood glucose emergency. Second, it's an excellent opportunity to spread awareness of the disease and perhaps educate them in the process. And finally, if your employer has allowed you extra breaks and other adjustments to check your glucose levels and treat yourself, letting colleagues in on the reason why can prevent feelings of ill will.

Your local Citizens Advice Bureau can also help you with further information about the Disability Discrimination Act and how it might protect you from discrimination at work.

Eat, Drink and Be Wary

Birthday parties, family reunions, wedding receptions, holidays, office gatherings – any event where food and drink play a starring role is a potential danger zone without the right preparation. If you know that the fare will be high in fat or sugar-rich, bring along a healthy dish (your host will probably appreciate the contribution anyway). Having a small snack at home before going to the event can help to blunt your appetite against too many temptations.

Don't forget that dancing is exercise. Check your glucose levels if you've been out on the dance floor for a while, to ensure that they aren't dropping too low. If food won't be available at all times during the party, bring a snack with you to fuel up with. A non-diet soda or juice from the bar can help to treat a hypo if you're caught without glucose tablets.

If you decide to enjoy beer, wine or a mixed drink, use caution and make sure you have a partner or friend with you who can recognize the signs of a hypo and treat them accordingly. See Chapter 14 for more on avoiding hypos when drinking.

Behind the Wheel

Having diabetes doesn't preclude you from driving, but it does mean that you have to take extra precautions, and there may be some legal restrictions placed upon you.

Always test before you drive, and if you're low, don't drive. Blood glucose levels below 4 mmol/l should be treated appropriately, and a safe blood glucose level should be attained before driving. If you start to experience symptoms of hypoglycaemia while you are driving, pull over immediately to test and treat. A hypo impairs your judgment and can cause you to lose consciousness. Like alcohol and falling asleep at the wheel, low blood glucose can easily result in a traffic fatality.

Diabetes UK point out that if you have a hypo while driving – and have an accident – you may be charged with driving under the influence of a drug (insulin), driving without due care and attention, or dangerous driving. Be safe – test your blood glucose levels and always take plenty of carbohydrate foods with you, even on short trips.

Licensing Issues

If you have diabetes that is treated with medication – tablets and/or insulin – by law you must inform the Driver and Vehicle Licensing Agency (DVLA). If your diabetes is treated by diet and exercise with no prescribed medication, you do not need to inform the DVLA – however, if you do start on tablets or insulin, you must inform them straight away. You must also inform the DVLA if you develop any complications of diabetes. If you ride a motorcycle, the rules for informing the DVLA about your diabetes are the same as those for people driving a car.

> You must inform your insurance company of your diabetes; failure to do so could invalidate a claim. Failure to inform the DVLA could also invalidate your cover.

People with diabetes who have complications, or who take insulin, must renew their licence every 1–3 years. The DVLA will send you the appropriate forms to be filled in in advance of your licence expiring. Getting your new licence may take a few weeks, especially if they need to contact your doctor or diabetes specialist for advice.

If your old licence expires before you receive your new one, ask your doctor if she considers you safe to drive – if this is the case, you are legally entitled to drive under Section 88 of the Road Traffic Act. However, if your previous licence was revoked for medical reasons, you must wait for your new licence to be issued.

Your motor insurance policy is protected by the DDA – insurers can only charge more or refuse cover if they have evidence of increased risk.

On a Road Trip

Taking a trip by car brings its own unique set of challenges to people living with diabetes. Prolonged sitting, road fatigue, fast-food dining and should-have-turned-left-at-the-last-exit-but-won't-ask-for-directions syndrome are just a few of the hazards you may have to overcome.

Stop and stretch often to get your circulation going and cut fatigue. It's a good idea to check your glucose levels at each rest stop as well. Again, pack snacks just in case you get waylaid or in case the next restaurant is far away. A cooler is an excellent idea if you're travelling in remote areas. A mobile phone is also essential for rural travel in case a breakdown leaves you stranded or you have a medical emergency.

Make sure all insulin, testing kits and medication are stored where they won't get excessively hot or cold. Boots, glove compartments and dashboards are all bad spots to keep your supplies. If you're in hot weather and you stop for a food or road break, do not leave your supplies and/or medication in the car unless you have a cooler to store them in. On a 23°C (73°F) day, in just ten minutes temperatures can reach 37°C (100°F) in a car with the windows closed, which will make your insulin go bad and possibly damage your meter and other equipment.

Be Prepared

However you travel, there are some basics you should carry with you at all times along with your toothbrush and clean underwear. These include:

- A first-aid kit, including antibiotic ointment and bandages
- Extra medication and insulin
- Blood glucose meter with double test strips and lancets
- Extra batteries for your meter and/or spare meter
- Emergency supply of fast-acting glucose
- Extra pump supplies (if applicable)
- Plenty of snacks, including fast-acting carbohydrates.

Always travel with twice the amount of medication and/or insulin you would normally require for the time you'll be gone. The same goes for blood glucose testing supplies. If you are delayed, your foresight will save you having to get a prescription filled in an unfamiliar place.

A sturdy, watertight supply case is a must for anyone who travels frequently. For those who take insulin, having a case that is well padded and insulated to keep vials or pens at their proper temperature is also important.

Travel Tips for the Wise

Holidays and business travel can present some unique control challenges and safety issues. Don't travel completely alone unless you have to. In case of an emergency, a trusted friend, partner or companion will be invaluable, particularly if you're in a foreign country. If you're a free spirit and like to go solo, make sure you always carry your basic medical information (i.e. name, diagnosis, medication, doctor contact) on your person, and wear your medical ID prominently.

Sea cruises are notorious for lavish buffets and total indulgence, but that doesn't mean you have to miss the boat. There are a growing number of cruise packages designed just for people with diabetes – with healthy and delicious cuisine, diabetes education and plenty of fun in the sun built into the itinerary. Talk to a travel agent.

Leisure Travellers

How many times have you returned from a holiday to feel more exhausted and burned out than before you left? Try to lose the 'hurry up and have fun – we're paying for this!' attitude and take a trip that involves actual rest and relaxation.

If you're travelling for leisure, try to throw strict schedules (except for those involving food and medication) out of the window. Stress can drive your blood glucose levels up and put a damper on your fun. Don't overplan your days, leave room for flexibility and enjoy just being in a new environment or culture.

Business Travellers

Travelling for business may throw some unexpected restrictions into your routine. A meeting with a client or an all-day workshop, and suddenly you find yourself behind schedule and going hypo. You can't work effectively if you don't take care of yourself, so excuse yourself if things run for longer than expected. In fact, the best approach is probably to mention a departure time as soon as your meeting begins, and stick to it. If you feel uncomfortable mentioning that you need a time out to eat or take medication due to your diabetes, then tell your client or colleague you have a dinner or lunch meeting to make (which is entirely true). You can also continue your business over a meal.

Many airlines offer meals for special diets, including 'diabetic' meals. Diabetes UK, however, advises against ordering these, as they are often low-carbohydrate meals. Instead, they recommend that you accept the standard meal and go with your own supply of fruit and biscuits and ask for extra bread to be available for you.

Air Travel and Medical Devices

In the last few years, air travel security measures have changed greatly in the UK and abroad. Because having diabetes necessitates travelling with medical sharps, there are some extra steps you may need to take to ensure you have easy access to your insulin and testing supplies while flying.

- **Insulin.** Keep all original packaging and paperwork that come with your insulin so you can present the original printed pharmaceutical label for the medication at the airport security checkpoint. The same applies for Glucagon kits. Syringes will be allowed past security only if the accompanying medication is properly labelled.
- **Meters.** You can take glucose meters and lancets in suitcases or hand baggage as long as meters are clearly marked with the manufacturer and/or brand name. Lancets should be capped and properly stored with the meter.
- **Pumps.** If you wear an insulin pump, inform airport security personnel and request so they can visually inspect it rather than removing it. Again, have insulin documentation with you. If screeners insist you remove your insulin pump, ask to speak to a security checkpoint supervisor.
- **Letter.** A letter from your doctor saying that you have diabetes and need to carry lancets, insulin, syringes, needles and/or pump supplies is a useful back-up.

Allow plenty of extra time for getting through airport security. You may want to plan on an extra 30–60 minutes in addition to whatever your airline is advising for advance arrival time. This will give you breathing room if airport personnel need to check your medical supplies. And always call the airline you'll be travelling with first to find out their specific security policies for the flight itself.

> If you have peripheral vascular disease, you run the risk of developing deep-vein thrombosis (DVT, or blood clotting) if you remain immobile for long periods of time. When you take a long flight or drive, make sure to get up and stretch your legs periodically. Wearing elastic compression stockings (i.e. support stockings) may also be beneficial. Make sure you check with your doctor before taking aspirin on a long-haul flight.

Adjusting Insulin and Time Zones

International travel requires some extra planning, particularly if you take insulin. In addition to the usual jet lag, you have to keep on schedule with your medication. In general, the easiest and most practical approach is to take insulin on track with meals in the 'new' time zone you're travelling in (or are en route to). However, you should always consult your doctor or diabetes specialist nurse about appropriate adjustments to insulin and medication before you travel, as the advice may vary based on the type of insulin you take, the distance you are travelling and other factors specific to your situation.

Staying Well Abroad

To stay healthy and safe while travelling in a foreign country, you should make sure you can communicate your needs adequately and are well supplied for the journey. Some tips:

· **Get your injections.** Before you go, make sure any required immunizations are up to date.

- **Learn the language.** If you don't speak the native tongue, make sure you have a guidebook to help you with basic medical phrases such as 'I need a doctor' and 'I have diabetes'.
- **Have your papers in order.** Keep your doctor's name and phone number along with your written insulin schedule on you at all times, and, as always, wear your medical identification.
- **Drink water.** If the water is questionable, drink bottled water (and don't put ice in any tinned and bottled beverages you order) to avoid diarrhoea or more serious illnesses.
- **Keep a food supply.** Make sure you have a stash of non-perishable snacks such as peanut butter and crackers, tinned fruit juice, raisins, dried apricots, nutrition bars and other foods that keep well and will serve as a mini-meal should your plans be interrupted.
- **Check your insurance.** Most travel insurance policies exclude pre-existing medical conditions – such as diabetes. If this is the case, you may not be covered for diabetes-related conditions, including heart attack or stroke. You might need to shop around; remember to check the small print carefully.

A number of diabetes drugs may cause photosensitivity (increased skin sensitivity to the sun) in those who use them. To minimize your risk, wear a brimmed hat and sunscreen with an SPF of 35 or higher for all exposed skin. Long sleeves and trouser legs also increase protection.

Chapter 22

Search for a Cure

Diabetes is, at present, an incurable disease. Although Type 2 diabetes can be well controlled to the point of normal or near-normal blood glucose levels, once you have it, it's a lifelong companion. While Type 1 diabetes can conceivably be 'cured' with a pancreas or islet transplant, both of these procedures currently require a lifelong regimen of immunosuppressive drugs. Still, great strides in genetics, transplantation techniques and stem cell research have brought a cure closer than ever.

A Short History

Diabetes was a death sentence for thousands of years until the discovery and isolation of insulin in 1921 provided the first groundbreaking step towards a cure. Before Sir Frederick Banting and Charles Best isolated the hormone, and colleagues J.J.R. Macleod and J.B. Collip helped purify and produce it for human use, the only treatment for diabetes was a near-starvation diet that resulted in slow wasting and eventual death.

Once insulin provided a way to treat the symptoms of diabetes, the challenge in the years that have followed has been to find a way to restore the insulin-producing capacity of the pancreas.

Collectively, genes dictate how cells grow and develop, as well as how they work and interact with each other. Individually, genes specify the production of individual proteins. If you know that a certain gene is at fault in a certain disease, you can study the gene to see what its function is, and this will give you clues as to what has gone wrong in the disease.

Genetic Discoveries

Numerous teams across the UK, and around the world, are busy researching the genetics of both Type 1 and Type 2 diabetes. An area of particular interest is the specific genes involved in maturity-onset diabetes in the young (MODY). Several genes have been identified that have then been isolated and studied in detail; this has enabled researchers to start to build up a picture of the various pathways involved in the growth and development of beta cells, and how they function to produce insulin.

Researchers are now using new knowledge of how beta cells in the pancreas are formed, in order to program non-specialized body cells (stem cells) to grow into insulin-producing beta cells. The ultimate hope is that stem cell research may lead to a cure for diabetes. (There is more on stem cell research later in this chapter.)

Unlocking the Beta Cell

Beta cells are the insulin-secreting cells of the pancreas. They are contained within islets (or islets of Langerhans) – cell clusters found within the pancreas. Islets are responsible for producing glucagon (alpha cells), insulin (beta cells), somatostatin (delta cells) and pancreatic peptide (PP cells). Destruction of the insulin-producing beta cells results in Type 1 diabetes, so the search for a cure has focused on finding a healthy replacement for these cells.

Islet transplantation has been under development since 1976, when the first successful animal islet transplant was performed by Dr. Paul Lacy, a JDRF (Juvenile Diabetes Research Foundation)-funded researcher.

Pancreas Transplants

One way to replace beta cell function and re-establish insulin independence is through a pancreas transplant. The procedure, however, is technically difficult and not performed that often in the UK. As of 1 April 2004, pancreas transplants for the residents of England are commissioned and funded by the Department of Health under the auspices of the National Specialist Commissioning Advisory Group (NSCAG). Seven centres in England have been designated by NSCAG to carry out pancreas transplants. Residents of Wales may be treated in England. Another centre, in Edinburgh, is commissioned by NHS Scotland.

A pancreas transplant can relieve your dependence on insulin, effectively curing you of diabetes; however, the immunosuppressive drugs that are required after a transplant can impose a new set of health problems. Because of the nasty side effects that the anti-rejection drugs can have, pancreas transplants tend to be restricted to people who are already in need of the immunosuppression – usually because they are having a kidney transplant at the same time, or they have already had a successful kidney transplant and are therefore already taking the drugs.

Isolated pancreas transplantation is performed occasionally, in people who suffer life-threatening hypoglycaemic unawareness.

Organs for transplant are still in much greater demand than supply. According to the Juvenile Diabetes Research Foundation (JDRF), for every 1 million people with Type 1 diabetes, there are only about 2,000 donor pancreases available each year for transplants.

Islet Transplants

Since only 2 per cent of the pancreas is composed of islets, a transplant of islets only is less invasive and has a much quicker recovery time than a full pancreas transplant. The Edmonton Protocol is a procedure for transplanting pancreatic islets into people with Type 1 diabetes in an effort to reverse their diabetes. The procedure, which was developed at the University of Alberta (Canada), involves infusing healthy, insulin-producing islets into the portal vein through a catheter. They are carried through the bloodstream to the liver, where they attach and begin functioning. The Edmonton Protocol also involves treating the patient post-transplant with a specialized steroid-free immunosuppressive cocktail of the drugs daclizumab, tacrolimus and sirolimus.

Dr James Shapiro, the lead researcher behind the Edmonton Protocol, first published the protocol and its remarkable success rates in the American *New England Journal of Medicine* in 2000. Since that time, clinical trials of the procedure have expanded rapidly and are taking place in the UK. At the time of publication of this book, researchers were reporting one-year success rates (as measured by insulin independence) of over 80 per cent, a significant advance over the dismal pre-Edmonton rates of less than 10 per cent.

One of the major obstacles in widespread application of islet transplantation is an inadequate supply of islets. The Edmonton protocol involves infusion of a larger volume of freshly harvested islets than previous islet transplantation methods used. In fact, two donated cadaver pancreases are required for each islet transplant procedure. Given the shortage of donated organs in the UK and abroad, this is where stem cell research may hold a prominent role in the search for a cure. In addition, there are numerous complications that could possibly occur as a result of islet transplantation, including bleeding, blood clots, gallbladder injury, worsening of lipids, elevation of blood pressure, worsening of kidney function, acne and mouth ulcers. Some of these complications are due to the procedure, while others are a result of the drugs being used.

Stem Cell Research

Stem cells are uncoded, 'generic' cells from which virtually all tissues of the body develop. These blank slates can be programmed into any organ tissue type, or blood cell, with the right set of genetic influences, or expressions.

The stem cells that have shown the most promise in diabetes research are those derived from in vitro fertilization (IVF), which are more commonly known as *embryonic stem cells*. These cells have the unique capacity to become any type of cell, tissue or organ as they mature and develop, yet they cannot themselves develop into a full human being. The feature that makes them most useful as a source for islets is that they can replicate themselves while remaining in an immature, or 'undifferentiated' state, thus offering a potentially unlimited source of cells for organ transplantation.

Growing Stem Cells

Stem cells are grown, or cultured, in a laboratory. The cells grow in a culture dish treated with a growth medium. The culture is sometimes treated with embryonic skin cells from mice, called feeder cells, to prevent the stem cells from dividing (or differentiating) and to provide nutrients to the culture. Because of the possibility of virus transmittal between human stem cells and feeder cells, researchers have been attempting to move away from this method of culturing cells.

Once cells have been cultured many times over, usually over the course of six months or longer, and have continued to reproduce without dividing or differentiating, they are said to be an established stem cell line, the basic materials that researchers use for specific experimentation.

A Matter of Controversy

Of course, stem cell research has become a political, social and ethical issue in the past decade because of the nature of embryonic stem cells. These cells are derived from a blastocyst – a hollow ball of cells from a four- or five-day-old embryo derived from an egg fertilized outside the body in an IVF clinic. The situation with respect to research on embryonic stem cells varies considerably across Europe. In the UK and several other countries, the research is allowed, while in other countries embryos are protected as human beings by law and, in some cases (including the Republic of Ireland) by the constitution. In the USA, federal funding and research is limited to a small number of existing cell lines.

Adult stem cells are a less controversial but, thus far, less productive area of diabetes research. These undifferentiated cells come from bone marrow or other areas of the body and act as a built-in first-aid kit, repairing tissue injury in the body. Scientists have also found that some of these adult stem cells can be coaxed into new tissues and organs.

Building a Better Pancreas

One goal of current diabetes research is to find a way to 'close the loop' on glucose monitoring and insulin treatment. In layperson's terms, this means a device that will monitor glucose levels and deliver insulin in response without any required operator intervention. Basically, this device would act as an artificial pancreas.

One closed-loop system currently in development is the long-term sensor system, or LTSS (Medtronic MiniMed), which is a surgically placed system that links an implantable long-term glucose sensor with an implantable insulin pump. The glucose sensor is implanted in the superior vena cava, a blood vessel near the heart, where it continuously monitors blood glucose levels. The sensor then transmits the information to the insulin pump, implanted in the abdomen, which in turn infuses the correct amount of insulin. The unit is programmed with a computerized device that uses radio frequency signals to send messages to the pump.

The LTSS requires an insulin refill every several months, which can be performed in a simple outpatient procedure using a syringe device. Safety mechanisms prevent the insulin from releasing unless it locks onto the correct port of the pump.

Another less-invasive version of a closed-loop system, in development by insulin pump manufacturer Disetronic, uses an external approach instead of an implantable one. The unit consists of a blood glucose sensor that adheres to the skin, an insulin pump and a small computer that analyzes glucose levels and signals the pump to infuse insulin in correct amounts in response. Medtronic MiniMed and Disetronic have artificial pancreas products in clinical trials, and predict bringing them to the market by 2007.

Clinical Trials

Clinical trials are scientific research studies that examine different aspects of a disease or medical condition or evaluate new drugs and other treatments. By participating in a clinical trial, you can get free access to new therapies not yet available to others. However, you also take any risks associated with an unproven treatment.

Clinical trials of new drugs fall into four different 'phase' categories. Phase 1 studies are initial, small-scale trials that help establish a safe dose and determine side effects. Phase 2 uses a larger study population at the dose established in phase 1 to determine the efficacy of the drug, and phase 3 and 4 studies compare the new drug with existing treatments for the same condition or illness.

All clinical trials are now subject to a new European Union directive that was implemented in UK law on 1 May 2004 (Medicines for Human Use

(Clinical Trials) Regulations 2004). The Medicines and Healthcare products Regulatory Agency (MHRA) is now the official regulatory body that oversees Good Clinical Practice and 'pharmacovigilance' in clinical trials. The new regulations clarify specific legal roles and responsibilities of sponsors, investigators and participants so the study design and protocol meet agreed specific ethical, clinical and safety standards.

Informed Consent

When you agree to participate in a clinical trial, you may not necessarily receive the treatment that the study is evaluating. Depending on the design of the study, you may be chosen to be part of a control group (a group of study subjects that does not receive the therapy being tested in order to serve as a baseline for comparison), or you may receive a placebo (an inactive substance that is sometimes administered to half of the study group, to measure the effectiveness of the treatment against a control).

Learning all of the potential ins and outs of a clinical trial is part of receiving informed consent on the study. Because the treatments examined in clinical trials are still experimental, informed consent is an important aspect of meeting the ethical guidelines of scientific study.

If you're interested in participating in a clinical trial, your first step is to check and see what is available. Diabetes UK is a good place to start. If you live near a teaching hospital or university, you can also check on available clinical trials there. Eligibility requirements will vary with each study.

It bears repeating yet again that the onset of Type 2 diabetes can be dramatically delayed or even halted with relatively minor lifestyle changes. If you are at risk for Type 2 diabetes but have not developed the condition yet, the best thing you can do for your health is to get on an exercise and healthy dietary programme.

Diabetes Prevention Program (DPP)

DPP was a landmark US study of 3,234 people with prediabetes (impaired glucose tolerance). The study found that diet and exercise slashed the risk of developing Type 2 diabetes by 58 per cent. The amount of exercise was just 30 minutes of moderate-intensity walking or similar workout routine daily, and the average weight loss was 5–7 per cent of body weight. The study also found that subjects with prediabetes who were given treatment with metformin reduced their risk of getting Type 2 diabetes by 31 per cent.

Diabetes Prevention Trial – Type 1 (DPT-1)

DPT-1 is a large-scale US study involving over 80,000 subjects who are considered 'at risk' of developing the disease (i.e. first- and second-degree relatives of people with Type 1 diabetes). The trial was still under way as at the publication of this book. However, one arm of the study, which looked at the effectiveness of low-dose insulin injections in preventing or delaying the onset of Type 1 diabetes in individuals considered high risk (i.e. greater than a 50 per cent chance of developing diabetes) was completed in 2002. Unfortunately, the DPT-1 found that insulin jabs were an ineffective preventative measure at the dose tested in high-risk individuals.

Phase two of DPT-1 is now exploring the possibility of whether oral insulin can prevent Type 1 diabetes in people at moderate risk (i.e. 25–50 per cent) of developing Type 1 diabetes within five years.

Advocacy Groups

You have the power of literally millions on your side in the fight against diabetes. Along with the 1.4 million other people with diabetes in the UK, Diabetes UK is fighting each day for diabetes rights, treatment advances, an end to discrimination and permanent solutions to diabetes.

Diabetes research also has many friends in Westminster, including MPs and representatives who have personally been touched by the disease. By adding your voice to the call for increases in research funding, both through your vote and with your support of advocacy and education in your community, you take the cause a little bit further. Yes, diabetes is a powerful enemy, but with strength in numbers, the fight can be won.

Appendix A

Additional Resources

General Diabetes Information (UK)

Diabetes UK *www.diabetes.org.uk*

Diabetes UK Careline email *careline@diabetes.org.uk*; tel 020 7424 1030

Diabetes UK Publications, tel 0800 585 088

Diabetes Insight *www.diabetes-insight.info*

General Diabetes Information (International)

About Diabetes at About.com hosted by Paula Ford-Martin *www.diabetes.about.com*

Dr Ian Blumer's Practical Guide to Diabetes *www.ianblumer.com*

Rick Mendosa's Diabetes Directory *www.mendosa.com*

Children with Diabetes (UK)

British Society for Paediatric Endocrinology and Diabetes *www.bsped.org.uk*

Juvenile Diabetes Research Foundation *www.jdrf.org.uk*

Children with Diabetes (International)

Children with Diabetes *www.childrenwithdiabetes.org*

Complications (UK)

British Heart Foundation *www.bhf.org.uk*

The Stroke Association *www.stroke.org.uk*

British Hypertension Society *www.hyp.ac.uk*

National Kidney Federation *www.kidney.org.uk*

The Neuropathy Trust *www.neuropathy-trust.org*

Sexual Dysfunction Association *www.sda.uk.net*

Royal National Institute for the Blind (RNIB) *www.rnib.org.uk*

Society for Chiropodists and Podiatrists *www.feetforlife.org*

Depression (UK)

Depression Alliance *www.depressionalliance.org*

The Samaritans *www.samaritans.org.uk*

Discrimination Issues (UK)

Disability Rights Commission *www.drc.org.uk*

Diabetes Discrimination in Employment *www.users.globalnet.co.uk/~irfduk*

Support Groups (UK)

Diabetes UK Voluntary Groups *www.diabetes.org.uk*

Diabetes Support *www.diabetes-insight.info*

The Children with Diabetes (US) website includes an email support group for UK parents of children with diabetes, accessible via the website. For more information on the UK group, email the list manager Jackie Jacombs *jackie.jacombs@childrenwithdiabetes.com*

Health Care (UK)

Department of Health *www.dh.gov.uk*

National Institute for Clinical Excellence *www.nice.org.uk*

Association of Community Health Councils for England and Wales *www.achcew.org.uk*

NHS Direct Online *www.nhsdirect.nhs.uk*

Patients Association *www.patients-association.com*

Research Information (UK)

Juvenile Diabetes Research Foundation *www.jdrf.org.uk*

Diabetes Genes *www.ex.ac.uk/diabetesgenes*

UK Children's Diabetes Research *www.childhood-diabetes.org.uk*

Travel (UK)

Diabetes Travel Information *www.diabetes-travel.co.uk*

Insulin Pumps (UK)

Insulin Pumpers UK *www.insulin-pumpers.org.uk*

Insulin Pump Therapy Group (INPUT) *www.webshowcase.net*

Diabetes Advocacy Organizations (International)

American Diabetes Association *www.diabetes.org*

Canadian Diabetes Association *www.diabetes.ca*

International Diabetes Federation (IDF) *www.idf.org*

European Association for the Study of Diabetes (EASD) *www.easd.org*

Other Organizations (UK)

British Ethnic Health Awareness Foundation (BHAF) *www.behaf.org.uk*

Eating Disorders Association (EDA) *www.edauk.com*

Verity (Polycystic Ovarian Syndrome) *www.verity-pcos.org.uk*

Other Organizations (International)

International Diabetic Athletes Association *www.diabetes-exercise.org*

Appendix B

Glucose Conversion Charts

HbA1c to Mean Daily Plasma Glucose Conversion

Use the following chart to work out how your HbA1c results convert to an average daily blood glucose reading.

HbA1c percentile	Average plasma glucose level in mg/dl	Average plasma glucose level in mmol/l
12.0 per cent	345	19.5
11.0 per cent	310	17.5
10.0 per cent	275	15.5
9.0 per cent	240	13.5
8.0 per cent	205	11.5
7.0 per cent	170	9.5
6.0 per cent	135	7.5
5.0 per cent	100	5.5
4.0 per cent	65	3.5

Recommended haemoglobin HbA1c goal from the American Association of Clinical Endocrinologists is ≤6.5 per cent; the American Diabetes Association recommends <7 per cent.

Conversion calculation based on Rohlfing CL, Wiedmeyer HM, Little RR, England JD, Tennill A, Goldstein DE: 'Defining the relationship between plasma glucose and HbA$_{1c}$: analysis of glucose profiles and HbA$_{1c}$ in the Diabetes Control and Complications Trial.' *Diabetes Care* 25:275–278, 2002.

Other Blood Glucose Conversions

In most countries, blood glucose is measured in mmol/l; however in the Unites States, blood glucose levels are measured in mg/dl. To convert between mg/dl and mmol/l:

1 mmol/l = 18 mg/dl
1 mg/dl = .055 mmol/l

To convert from plasma to whole blood:

Plasma readings run about 15 per cent higher than whole-blood readings. Equation conversion factor: plasma = whole blood ˘ 1.12

Index